Independent RNC-OB Exam Prep 2027–2028:

750 Practice Questions with Domain-Based Review and Detailed Explanations for NCC Inpatient Obstetric Nurse

Abiodun Caldwell

STUDY GUIDE BONUS MATERIAL

Full Audio Edition

Access the complete book in audio format
Ideal for learning during travel, workouts, or downtime
Stay productive even when you're not in the mood to read

Digital Flashcards

Fast and effective revision tool
Strengthen memory of important concepts
Study anytime, wherever you are

Quick & Easy Access

No sign-up needed
Compatible with all devices
Smooth and instant usability

Access all bonus content on Page 17

Author Introduction

Registered Nurse Certified (RNC) credentialing represents a professional milestone for nurses who are committed to advancing clinical excellence, demonstrating specialized competence, and elevating standards of patient care. Preparing for this certification demands more than memorization; it requires clinical judgment, analytical precision, and the ability to apply evidence-based knowledge in complex healthcare environments. This study guide was developed with that challenge in mind.

The author of this guide is an experienced nursing educator and clinician who has dedicated a career to supporting professional nurses in achieving certification success. Working in collaboration with a focused team of nurse educators, subject-matter specialists, and clinical reviewers, the author has helped design comprehensive preparation strategies aligned with the competencies assessed in Registered Nurse Certified examinations. Together, this team has analyzed exam blueprints, reviewed current standards of practice, and integrated the latest evidence-based guidelines to ensure this resource reflects the rigor and relevance of today's nursing profession.

With years of experience mentoring candidates across diverse specialties, the author understands the realities facing working nurses: demanding schedules, evolving clinical protocols, and the pressure to balance professional growth with patient responsibilities. This insight shapes the structure of the guide, which emphasizes clarity, efficiency, and practical application. Rather than overwhelming readers with unnecessary detail, the material focuses on high-yield concepts, clinical reasoning frameworks, and test-taking strategies specifically tailored to certification-level assessment.

Every chapter is organized to strengthen both foundational knowledge and higher-order thinking skills. Practice questions mirror the format and cognitive demands of certification exams, encouraging nurses to think critically, prioritize patient safety, and apply standards of care with confidence. Detailed rationales reinforce understanding and help bridge the gap between theory and real-world clinical decision-making.

Above all, this guide reflects a commitment to professional excellence and lifelong learning. Certification is not merely an examination—it is a declaration of competence, dedication, and leadership within the nursing field. The author and contributing team share a unified mission: to equip nurses with the tools, confidence, and strategic insight necessary to approach the Registered Nurse Certified examination with assurance and to emerge prepared not only to pass, but to excel in their practice.

Table of Contents

The information contained in this publication is provided for educational and informational purposes. While every effort has been made to ensure accuracy, completeness, and relevance at the time of publication, the author and contributing team make no representations or warranties regarding the completeness or suitability of the content for any specific purpose. Readers are encouraged to consult official exam resources and governing bodies for the most current policies, procedures, and requirements related to certification.

This publication is not affiliated with, endorsed by, or sponsored by any official certifying organization. All product names, trademarks, and registered trademarks referenced herein are the property of their respective owners.

The author and publisher disclaim any liability for any direct, indirect, incidental, consequential, or other damages arising from the use of this material. By using this guide, the reader agrees to these terms.

Disclaimer

RNC-OB® is a registered trademark of National Certification Corporation. This publication is an independent study tool and is not affiliated with or endorsed by NCC.

Chapter 1: Pregnancy Complications, Treatment, and Management

Understanding Maternal-Fetal Complexity

Pregnancy is a profound physiologic transformation that challenges nearly every maternal organ system while simultaneously supporting the continuous growth and development of a genetically distinct individual within the uterus. This process is not static but highly dynamic, requiring constant adaptation as maternal physiology evolves across each trimester to meet the increasing metabolic and oxygen demands of the fetus. The dynamic equilibrium that maintains this state is inherently delicate, relying on finely tuned regulatory mechanisms that integrate cardiovascular, endocrine, renal, hematologic, and metabolic functions. Even minor disruptions in this balance can initiate a cascade of events that lead to complications with significant and sometimes life-threatening implications for both the mother and the fetus. Understanding pregnancy as a shared adaptive process allows clinicians to interpret pathologic changes not as isolated failures of a single system, but rather as breakdowns in the complex physiologic coordination that normally sustains maternal–fetal well-being.

From a systems perspective, pregnancy requires the maternal body to operate at an enhanced functional capacity. The cardiovascular system, for example, undergoes substantial remodeling, including marked expansion of plasma volume, increased cardiac output, and decreased systemic vascular resistance, all of which are essential to ensure adequate uteroplacental perfusion and optimal fetal oxygenation. At the same time, the endocrine system orchestrates hormonal changes involving progesterone, estrogen, human placental lactogen, and insulin, which collectively regulate metabolism, promote nutrient availability, and support fetal growth. The renal system adapts through increased glomerular filtration rate and altered fluid and electrolyte handling to maintain homeostasis in the face of expanded blood volume and metabolic waste production. These interdependent adjustments illustrate how pregnancy is sustained through coordinated physiologic recalibration rather than isolated organ function. However, when these compensatory mechanisms exceed their adaptive capacity or become dysregulated, pathologic conditions can emerge. Disorders such as preeclampsia reflect abnormal vascular adaptation and endothelial dysfunction, while gestational diabetes arises from impaired glucose metabolism and insulin resistance driven by placental hormones. Placental insufficiency, on the other hand, represents a failure of adequate placental perfusion and nutrient exchange, compromising fetal growth and development. These conditions highlight how breakdowns in physiologic integration can have multisystem consequences, reinforcing the importance of early recognition and comprehensive understanding.

Effective nursing management in obstetrics requires more than the ability to identify clinical signs and symptoms; it demands a deep comprehension of the underlying physiologic mechanisms that drive both normal adaptation and pathologic change. In high-acuity settings, maternal and fetal outcomes depend heavily on the nurse's capacity to anticipate complications before they fully manifest, interpret subtle deviations from normal patterns, and respond rapidly with appropriate interventions. This includes continuous assessment, critical thinking, and collaboration within interdisciplinary teams that integrate medical, surgical, and psychosocial approaches to care. The nurse must also consider the emotional and psychological dimensions of pregnancy, as stress and environmental factors can further influence physiologic stability. Ultimately, each pregnancy represents a unique physiologic dialogue between maternal reserves and fetal demands, shaped by genetic, environmental, and health-related factors. This dialogue is ongoing and requires vigilant monitoring to ensure that both participants in the maternal–fetal unit remain stable and supported. The nurse's role is to observe, interpret, and respond to this evolving interaction continuously, using clinical expertise to maintain balance, prevent deterioration, and promote optimal outcomes for both mother and child.

Hypertensive Disorders of Pregnancy

Table: Hypertensive Disorders Comparison

Condition	Key Features	Diagnostic Criteria	Complications
Gestational Hypertension	Elevated BP after 20 weeks	≥140/90 mmHg	May progress to preeclampsia
Preeclampsia	HTN + proteinuria	BP + ≥300 mg protein	Eclampsia, HELLP
Eclampsia	Seizures in preeclampsia	Convulsions	Maternal/fetal mortality
Chronic HTN	Pre-existing HTN	Before 20 weeks	Placental insufficiency

Hypertensive conditions are among the most serious complications affecting obstetric outcomes, encompassing gestational hypertension, preeclampsia, and eclampsia. These disorders represent systemic endothelial dysfunction leading to widespread vasospasm, reduced placental perfusion, and potential multiorgan compromise. The clinical picture may include elevated blood pressure, proteinuria, headache, visual disturbances, and epigastric pain. The nurse's vigilance is critical in recognizing subtle neurological or renal signs that herald disease progression. According to established obstetric literature, careful fluid management, controlled antihypertensive therapy, and seizure prophylaxis with magnesium sulfate form the core of stabilization. Continuous fetal assessment ensures that intrauterine compromise is detected early, guiding timely delivery decisions. Emotional support remains equally essential as these conditions often provoke fear and uncertainty. The obstetric nurse's calm presence and patient education on warning signs during hospitalization and postpartum recovery reduce anxiety and improve adherence to follow-up. Hypertensive disorders underscore the principle that maternal physiology can shift swiftly from adaptation to crisis, demanding both technical skill and compassionate communication from every clinician involved in care.

Hemorrhagic Emergencies and Placental Disorders

Hemorrhage remains a leading cause of maternal mortality worldwide, and prompt recognition of its sources is vital. Antepartum bleeding often results from placental abnormalities such as previa or abruption, while postpartum hemorrhage frequently stems from uterine atony, retained tissue, or genital tract trauma. The physiologic challenge of hemorrhage is twofold: preserving oxygen delivery to vital organs while sustaining uteroplacental perfusion. Clinical response requires simultaneous resuscitation, uterotonic administration, and surgical or procedural intervention if bleeding persists. The obstetric nurse plays a central role in early quantification of blood loss, coordination of transfusion protocols, and monitoring for coagulopathy. Texts in advanced obstetric practice highlight the importance of teamwork, structured communication, and use of checklists in preventing escalation. Modern strategies, including uterine balloon tamponade and rapid access to blood products, have transformed survival outcomes. Yet beyond technical measures, nurses safeguard psychological stability, supporting patients and families through moments of uncertainty. Hemorrhagic emergencies epitomize obstetric unpredictability and reaffirm the necessity of preparedness, vigilance, and structured post-event debriefing to sustain clinical resilience.

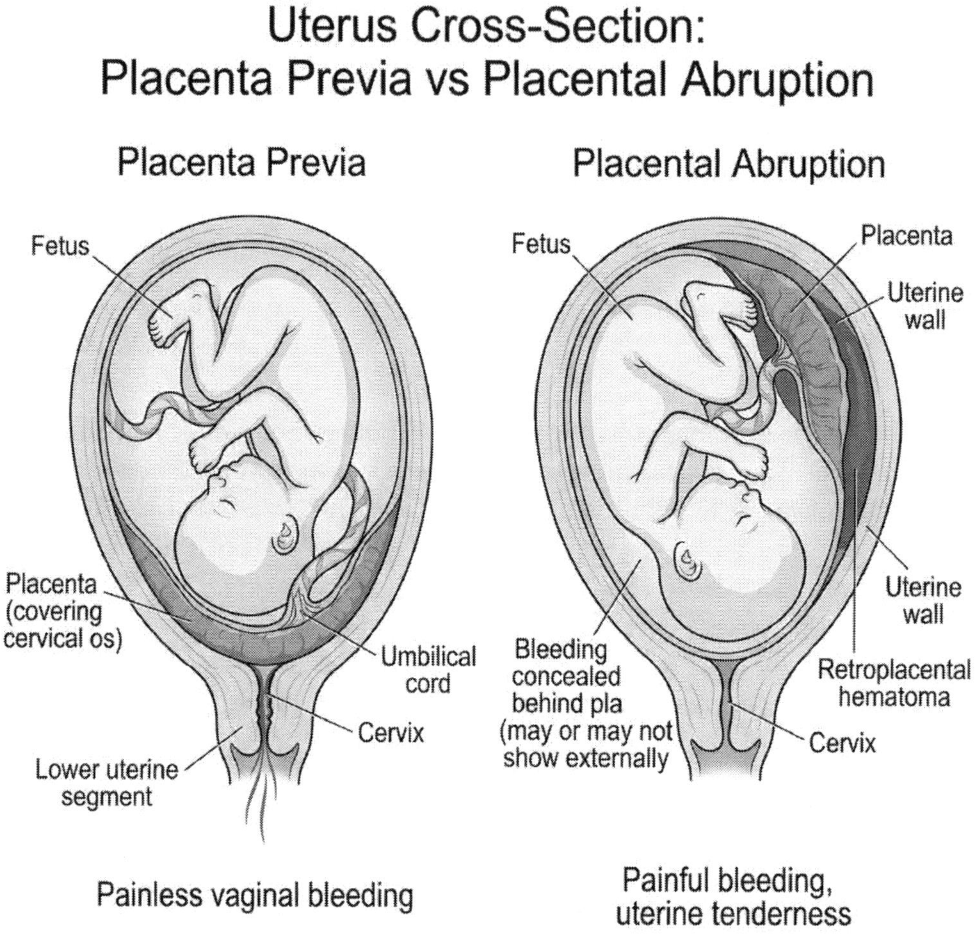

Endocrine and Metabolic Complications

Metabolic adaptations in pregnancy, although fundamentally protective and essential for supporting fetal growth and development, can paradoxically predispose individuals to a range of metabolic and endocrine disorders, most notably gestational diabetes mellitus and thyroid dysfunction. These adaptations are driven by the physiologic need to prioritize a continuous and adequate supply of nutrients to the fetus, even in conditions where maternal intake may fluctuate. As pregnancy progresses, maternal metabolism shifts from an anabolic state in early gestation, characterized by energy storage, to a catabolic state in later trimesters, where stored nutrients are mobilized to meet the increasing demands of the developing fetus. While this transition is necessary for fetal survival, it also places significant stress on maternal regulatory systems, increasing the likelihood that underlying vulnerabilities will manifest as clinical disease.

A central component of these metabolic changes is the role of the placenta as a highly active endocrine organ. The placenta produces a variety of hormones, including human placental lactogen, progesterone, estrogen, cortisol, and growth hormone–like substances, all of which contribute to the development of insulin resistance in maternal tissues. This insulin resistance is physiologically advantageous because it reduces maternal glucose utilization and ensures a steady supply of glucose to the fetus via facilitated diffusion across the placenta. However, when maternal pancreatic function is unable to compensate for this increased insulin demand through adequate insulin secretion, maternal hyperglycemia develops, resulting in gestational diabetes mellitus. This condition represents not merely an elevation in blood glucose levels, but a disruption in the delicate metabolic balance that normally supports pregnancy. The consequences of maternal hyperglycemia extend beyond the mother and have significant implications for fetal development. Elevated maternal glucose levels lead to increased transplacental glucose transfer, which stimulates fetal pancreatic insulin production. This hyperinsulinemic state promotes excessive fetal growth, or macrosomia, increasing the risk of complications such as shoulder dystocia, birth trauma, and operative delivery. After birth, the sudden interruption of maternal glucose supply can result in neonatal hypoglycemia due to persistent high insulin levels. Additionally, exposure to an intrauterine hyperglycemic environment has been associated with long-term metabolic consequences for the child, including an increased risk of obesity and type 2 diabetes later in life. These outcomes underscore the importance of early identification and meticulous management of gestational diabetes.

Nursing care in the context of gestational diabetes is multifaceted and requires a comprehensive approach to glucose regulation. This includes the implementation of individualized dietary planning aimed at controlling carbohydrate intake while ensuring adequate nutrition, as well as the promotion of regular physical activity to enhance insulin sensitivity. When lifestyle modifications are insufficient, pharmacologic interventions such as insulin therapy or oral hypoglycemic agents may be necessary, requiring careful monitoring and patient education to ensure safe and effective use. Continuous fetal surveillance is also a critical component of care, as it allows for the early detection of abnormalities in fetal growth and well-being. Techniques such as serial ultrasounds and assessment of fetal movement patterns help guide clinical decision-making and timing of delivery. In parallel, thyroid function plays a crucial role in maintaining normal pregnancy physiology, and disturbances in thyroid hormone levels can significantly impact both maternal health and fetal development. Hypothyroidism, in particular, is associated with adverse outcomes such as miscarriage, preterm birth, and impaired neurodevelopment in the fetus. Thyroid hormones are essential for fetal brain development, especially in early pregnancy before the fetal thyroid gland becomes fully functional. Therefore, inadequate maternal thyroid hormone levels during this critical period can have lasting effects on cognitive function and neurological maturation. Hyperthyroidism, although less common, also presents risks, including fetal growth restriction and maternal complications such as preeclampsia.

Managing thyroid disorders during pregnancy requires a precise balance of pharmacologic therapy and ongoing monitoring. Medications such as levothyroxine for hypothyroidism must be carefully titrated based on regular assessment of thyroid-stimulating hormone and free thyroxine levels, as physiologic changes in pregnancy alter hormone requirements. Equally important is patient-centered education, which emphasizes the necessity of strict medication adherence, timing of doses, and awareness of potential symptoms indicating inadequate or excessive treatment. The nurse plays a critical role in reinforcing this education, ensuring that patients understand both the rationale for therapy and the importance of consistent follow-up. The nurse also serves as a vital liaison between laboratory monitoring and the patient's lived experience, translating complex biochemical data into practical and understandable self-care strategies. This role involves not only interpreting laboratory values but also integrating them with clinical observations and patient-reported symptoms. Subtle changes in energy levels, appetite, weight, and overall well-being may provide early of metabolic imbalance, even before laboratory abnormalities become pronounced. By recognizing these early warning signs, nurses can facilitate timely intervention, preventing progression to more severe complications.

Furthermore, attention to fetal indicators, such as patterns of movement and growth, adds another layer of assessment that complements maternal monitoring. Encouraging patients to remain aware of fetal activity and to report any deviations from expected patterns empowers them to participate actively in their own care. This collaborative approach strengthens the therapeutic relationship and enhances the effectiveness of management strategies. Ultimately, successful management of metabolic and endocrine disorders in pregnancy depends on individualized vigilance rather than reliance on standardized routines. Each patient presents with a unique interplay of physiologic responses, risk factors, and lifestyle considerations that must be taken into account when developing a care plan. The nurse's role is to synthesize clinical knowledge, patient education, and ongoing assessment into a cohesive strategy that supports both maternal and fetal health. Through continuous monitoring, early recognition of abnormalities, and responsive intervention, nurses help maintain the delicate metabolic balance that is essential for a healthy pregnancy outcome.

Infectious and Immunologic Disorders

Pregnancy introduces a state of carefully regulated immunologic tolerance that permits the survival and growth of the fetus, which is genetically distinct from the mother, while simultaneously increasing maternal vulnerability to certain infections. This immunologic adaptation is not a simple suppression of the immune system but rather a complex modulation that shifts immune responses to favor tolerance over rejection. Cellular immunity, particularly T-cell–mediated responses, becomes selectively downregulated, while aspects of humoral immunity remain active. This balance allows the maternal body to coexist with fetal antigens without initiating an immune attack, yet it also reduces the body's ability to effectively combat specific intracellular pathogens. As a result, pregnant individuals may experience altered susceptibility, atypical symptom presentation, and increased severity of infections, all of which can significantly influence maternal health and perinatal outcomes.

Pathogens such as group B streptococcus, cytomegalovirus, and influenza are of particular concern in pregnancy due to their potential to cause serious complications for both the mother and the fetus. Group B streptococcus colonization, for instance, may be asymptomatic in the mother but can lead to neonatal sepsis, pneumonia, or meningitis if transmitted during labor and delivery. Cytomegalovirus, a common viral infection, poses a risk of congenital infection, which may result in long-term neurologic impairment, hearing loss, or developmental delays. Influenza infection during pregnancy is associated with increased risk of severe respiratory illness, hospitalization, and adverse fetal outcomes such as preterm birth. These examples highlight the critical importance of early identification, prevention, and management of infectious diseases in the obstetric population.

The obstetric nurse's expertise lies in the ability to recognize atypical or subtle presentations of infection, which may differ significantly from those observed in nonpregnant individuals. Symptoms such as mild fever, fatigue, or vague discomfort may be the only indicators of an underlying infectious process, requiring heightened clinical vigilance and critical thinking. Prompt initiation of appropriate isolation precautions, when indicated, is essential to prevent transmission within healthcare settings and to protect both patients and healthcare providers. In addition, timely administration of antimicrobial or antiviral therapy, guided by clinical protocols and laboratory findings, plays a crucial role in minimizing disease progression and improving outcomes. The nurse must also monitor for therapeutic effectiveness and potential side effects, ensuring that treatment remains both safe and effective throughout the course of care.

Global clinical guidelines emphasize the importance of preventive strategies, including vaccination, hygiene education, and routine screening protocols, to reduce the incidence of preventable infections during pregnancy. Vaccination against influenza and other recommended pathogens provides a critical layer of protection for both the mother and the fetus, while education on hand hygiene, food safety, and avoidance of infectious exposures empowers patients to actively participate in their own care. Screening programs, such as those for group B streptococcus, enable early identification and targeted intervention, reducing the risk of neonatal transmission and associated complications. These preventive measures are most effective when consistently implemented and reinforced through patient education and clinical practice. Beyond microbial threats, pregnancy also presents immunologic challenges related to conditions such as Rh incompatibility and autoimmune diseases. Rh incompatibility occurs when there is a mismatch between maternal and fetal blood types, leading to the potential development of maternal antibodies against fetal red blood cells. This immune response can result in hemolytic disease of the fetus and newborn, a condition that requires careful monitoring and, in some cases, intrauterine intervention. Autoimmune diseases, including conditions such as systemic lupus erythematosus, involve dysregulation of the immune system that can be further complicated by the physiologic changes of pregnancy. These disorders create complex clinical scenarios in which maternal and fetal immune interactions are closely intertwined, necessitating coordinated laboratory assessment, ongoing surveillance, and interdisciplinary management.

Effective management of these immunologic conditions requires a comprehensive approach that integrates laboratory data, clinical assessment, and fetal monitoring. Serial testing, including antibody titers and markers of disease activity, provides essential information for guiding treatment decisions. Intrauterine monitoring techniques, such as ultrasound and fetal well-being assessments, allow for early detection of complications and timely intervention. The nurse plays a central role in coordinating these aspects of care, ensuring that information is accurately communicated among healthcare providers and that interventions are implemented promptly. Equally important is the provision of emotional support and reassurance to patients, as the diagnosis of an infection or immunologic condition during pregnancy often evokes significant anxiety, fear, and feelings of guilt regarding potential harm to the fetus. Patients may struggle with uncertainty about outcomes and the implications of treatment, making compassionate communication an essential component of care. Through clear, consistent explanations and empathetic engagement, nurses help patients understand their condition, the rationale for interventions, and the steps being taken to protect both maternal and fetal health. This supportive approach not only alleviates emotional distress but also enhances patient adherence to treatment plans.

The nurse's role extends beyond clinical management to include advocacy, education, and the fostering of trust within the patient–provider relationship. By translating complex medical information into accessible language, nurses empower patients to participate actively in decision-making and self-care practices. Encouraging open communication and addressing patient concerns in a respectful and nonjudgmental manner further strengthens this partnership.

Infection control in pregnancy, therefore, extends far beyond the application of sterile technique or adherence to clinical protocols. It encompasses a holistic approach that includes maintaining patient confidentiality, protecting privacy, and creating an environment in which patients feel safe and supported. Promoting hope amid uncertainty is a vital aspect of this process, as it helps patients navigate the challenges of pregnancy complications with resilience and confidence. Ultimately, the management of immunologic and infectious conditions during pregnancy requires a balance of scientific knowledge, clinical skill, and compassionate care. By continuously monitoring for signs of infection, implementing preventive strategies, and addressing both the physical and emotional needs of patients, nurses play a pivotal role in safeguarding maternal and fetal well-being. Through individualized care and vigilant assessment, they help sustain the delicate immunologic balance that is essential for a successful pregnancy outcome.

Preterm Labor and Premature Rupture of Membranes

Preterm birth remains one of obstetrics' most pressing global challenges, representing a leading cause of neonatal morbidity and mortality worldwide and contributing significantly to long-term neurodevelopmental impairment in surviving infants. Defined by the onset of labor before thirty-seven weeks' gestation, preterm birth is not a singular condition but rather a multifactorial syndrome with diverse etiologies and clinical pathways. It may arise from intrauterine infection, which triggers inflammatory responses that stimulate uterine contractions, from uterine overdistention as seen in multifetal gestation or polyhydramnios, or from idiopathic causes in which no clear precipitating factor can be identified. This complexity underscores the difficulty in predicting and preventing preterm labor, as well as the necessity for vigilant monitoring throughout pregnancy.

The pathophysiology of preterm labor involves a cascade of biochemical and mechanical events that lead to cervical ripening, uterine contractility, and eventual delivery. Early rupture of membranes, particularly preterm premature rupture of membranes, further increases the risk for neonatal morbidity by exposing the fetus to ascending infections and reducing the protective barrier provided by amniotic fluid. This condition not only accelerates the onset of labor but also heightens the risk of complications such as chorioamnionitis, cord prolapse, and fetal distress. The interplay between infection, inflammation, and mechanical stress highlights the fragile balance that maintains pregnancy and the multiple points at which this balance can be disrupted. Effective management of preterm labor requires careful consideration of competing priorities, balancing the urgency of prolonging gestation to allow for further fetal maturation against the need to prevent maternal infection or fetal compromise. Clinical decision-making often involves determining whether continuation of the pregnancy poses greater risk than early delivery. Interventions are therefore tailored to the individual clinical scenario, taking into account gestational age, presence of infection, fetal status, and maternal condition. This dynamic process requires continuous reassessment and close collaboration among healthcare providers.

Nursing priorities in the management of preterm labor are both comprehensive and highly detail-oriented, beginning with accurate assessment of uterine activity, including frequency, duration, and intensity of contractions. Subtle changes in contraction patterns may represent early signs of preterm labor, requiring prompt recognition and intervention. Assessment of fluid leakage is equally critical, as it may indicate rupture of membranes, necessitating further evaluation and potential modification of the care plan. Monitoring cervical change through clinical examination or diagnostic tools provides additional information about labor progression and helps guide therapeutic decisions.

Pharmacologic management plays a key role in delaying preterm birth and improving neonatal outcomes. The administration of corticosteroids is a cornerstone of therapy, as it accelerates fetal lung maturation and reduces the risk of respiratory distress syndrome, intraventricular hemorrhage, and neonatal mortality. Tocolytic agents may be used to suppress uterine contractions temporarily, allowing time for corticosteroids to take effect or for transfer to a facility with appropriate neonatal care capabilities. The nurse is responsible for administering these medications safely, monitoring for side effects, and evaluating their effectiveness, all while maintaining clear communication with the healthcare team.

In addition to clinical interventions, continuous emotional support and patient education are essential components of care. The experience of preterm labor can be highly stressful and anxiety-provoking for patients, who may fear for the health and survival of their infant. Providing clear explanations of the condition, treatment options, and expected outcomes helps reduce uncertainty and empowers patients to participate actively in their care. Education regarding the importance of adherence to bed rest, medication regimens, and follow-up appointments enhances compliance and contributes to more favorable outcomes. Literature on high-risk pregnancy consistently emphasizes that nurses are often the first to recognize subtle signs of preterm activity, such as mild contractions, pelvic pressure, or changes in vaginal discharge. These early indicators may be easily overlooked but can signal the onset of significant physiologic changes. Through precise observation and attentive listening to patient concerns, nurses play a critical role in identifying these warning signs before they progress to more advanced stages of labor. This early recognition allows for timely intervention, which can be crucial in delaying delivery and improving neonatal prognosis.

Clear and thorough documentation is another essential aspect of nursing practice in this context, as it ensures continuity of care and facilitates effective communication among members of the healthcare team. Accurate recording of assessment findings, interventions, and patient responses provides a comprehensive picture of the patient's condition and supports informed clinical decision-making. Rapid communication of significant changes or concerns enables prompt action and reduces the risk of adverse outcomes. Preventive strategies also play a vital role in reducing the incidence of preterm birth and are an integral part of ongoing antenatal care. Counseling patients on adequate hydration helps maintain uterine relaxation and reduces the likelihood of contraction initiation. Education on infection prevention, including proper hygiene and timely treatment of urinary or vaginal infections, addresses one of the key modifiable risk factors for preterm labor. Lifestyle modifications, such as smoking cessation, stress reduction, and appropriate physical activity, further contribute to maintaining pregnancy health and stability.

Ultimately, the management of preterm birth exemplifies the intersection of clinical expertise, preventive care, and compassionate support. It demonstrates how knowledge and empathy converge in everyday nursing practice, allowing healthcare providers to address not only the physiologic aspects of preterm labor but also the emotional and psychological needs of patients. By combining vigilant assessment, evidence-based interventions, and patient-centered communication, nurses serve as the frontline defense against premature delivery, striving to optimize outcomes for both mother and infant.

Multifetal Gestation and Physiologic Adaptation

Carrying more than one fetus magnifies the physiological demands of pregnancy and introduces a distinct spectrum of risks. Increased uterine distention predisposes to preterm labor, malpresentation, and hemorrhage, while maternal cardiovascular workload intensifies substantially. Each additional fetus compounds nutritional and hemodynamic requirements, making meticulous monitoring indispensable.

The nurse's role extends from early education about nutritional adequacy to vigilant surveillance for hypertensive disorders and fetal growth discordance. Ultrasound evaluation, serial fundal measurements, and individualized rest schedules become routine. Communication among the care team must remain seamless as complications can evolve abruptly. Beyond medical vigilance, emotional care holds equal weight, as families often experience heightened anxiety and logistical stress. Practical guidance on hospital preparedness, newborn care planning, and postpartum support helps transform anxiety into empowerment. Multifetal pregnancy illustrates both the marvel and fragility of human reproduction, underscoring the nurse's function as stabilizer, educator, and advocate through every unpredictable turn.

Psychological and Environmental Influences

Pregnancy unfolds within complex emotional and social contexts that profoundly affect maternal health. Stress, domestic violence, financial instability, and inadequate support can heighten vulnerability to complications. The physiological stress response—mediated by cortisol and catecholamines—can impair uteroplacental perfusion and influence labor outcomes. Effective nursing care integrates psychosocial screening into every clinical encounter, identifying depression, anxiety, or trauma that may otherwise remain invisible. The World Health Organization emphasizes compassionate communication and nonjudgmental listening as essential interventions, often as vital as medical treatment. Nurses foster trust by creating safe spaces where women feel heard and respected. Environmental exposures such as tobacco smoke, pollutants, or occupational hazards also demand assessment and education. Through holistic evaluation, the nurse becomes a guardian of both physical and emotional safety. Recognizing that health cannot be separated from circumstance transforms obstetric care into a human partnership grounded in empathy, advocacy, and cultural sensitivity.

Integrating Management and Interdisciplinary Collaboration

The successful management of pregnancy complications depends on collaboration that transcends professional boundaries. Obstetric nurses function within multidisciplinary teams that include physicians, anesthetists, neonatologists, social workers, and lactation consultants. Effective teamwork relies on shared situational awareness, structured communication, and mutual respect. Evidence from clinical quality initiatives shows that standardized response protocols, such as rapid obstetric emergency systems, reduce morbidity when nurses are empowered to activate them without hesitation. Integration also includes continuous education—simulation training, case reviews, and morbidity conferences refine collective readiness. The nurse's reflective practice closes the loop, transforming experience into insight and insight into safer care. As the first chapter of this guide concludes, one truth becomes clear: excellence in obstetric nursing arises not from solitary expertise but from coordinated vigilance. The complexity of pregnancy demands not isolated mastery but cooperative intelligence, sustained empathy, and unwavering dedication to the dual life entrusted to every caregiver.

Access Audio file and Flashcards

Scan QR Code Below

Chapter 2: Fetal Assessment

1. Foundations of Fetal Surveillance

Fetal assessment represents a vital intersection of physiology, ethics, and technology within obstetric care, encompassing far more than the simple measurement of fetal parameters. It reflects a comprehensive and ongoing effort to evaluate the condition of the fetus within the intrauterine environment, recognizing that fetal well-being is inseparably linked to maternal health and placental function. The fundamental goal of fetal assessment is to determine fetal well-being by evaluating oxygenation, growth, and the fetus's ability to adapt to changing uterine conditions. These elements are not static but evolve continuously throughout pregnancy and labor, requiring repeated evaluation and thoughtful interpretation. In this context, fetal assessment becomes a dynamic clinical process that integrates scientific knowledge with ethical responsibility, ensuring that both maternal and fetal interests are carefully balanced.

The concept of surveillance extends beyond the mere detection of fetal distress; it embodies a continuous and responsive dialogue between maternal physiology and fetal response. This dialogue is mediated through the placenta, which serves as the critical interface for gas exchange, nutrient delivery, and waste removal. The uterus functions as a dynamic environment where maternal blood flow, placental efficiency, and hormonal regulation interact to maintain a delicate equilibrium necessary for fetal survival. Any disruption in this balance—whether due to decreased uteroplacental perfusion, placental insufficiency, or maternal illness—can compromise fetal oxygenation and lead to adaptive or maladaptive responses. Recognizing these changes early through systematic and vigilant assessment becomes one of the nurse's highest responsibilities, as timely intervention can prevent progression to irreversible fetal compromise. A thorough understanding of fetal physiology forms the scientific foundation of all assessment techniques. Fetal heart rate regulation, for example, reflects the interplay between the autonomic nervous system and oxygenation status, providing critical insight into fetal well-being. Variability in heart rate indicates a functioning central nervous system and adequate oxygenation, while changes such as accelerations or decelerations may signal adaptation or distress. Similarly, acid–base homeostasis is a key indicator of fetal metabolic status, with hypoxia leading to anaerobic metabolism and the accumulation of lactic acid. The fetus's response to hypoxia, including compensatory mechanisms such as redistribution of blood flow to vital organs, illustrates the complexity of physiologic adaptation and underscores the importance of accurate interpretation of monitoring data.

Effective fetal surveillance relies on a combination of technological tools and clinical judgment. Techniques such as intermittent auscultation and continuous electronic fetal monitoring allow for the observation of fetal heart rate patterns in relation to uterine activity, providing valuable information about the fetus's response to labor . However, the presence of monitoring equipment alone does not ensure optimal care; it is the interpretation of these data within the broader clinical context that determines their value. Factors such as maternal condition, gestational age, risk status, and labor progression must all be considered when evaluating fetal status. This holistic approach ensures that clinical decisions are individualized and responsive to the unique circumstances of each patient. The professional nurse plays a central role in synthesizing these multiple dimensions into a coherent clinical picture that guides intervention, promotes comfort, and provides reassurance. This involves not only technical proficiency in operating monitoring but also critical thinking skills to analyze patterns, recognize deviations from normal, and anticipate potential complications. Clear communication with the healthcare team is essential to ensure that significant findings are addressed promptly and appropriately. At the same time, the nurse must communicate effectively with the patient, explaining procedures, findings, and implications in a manner that is both understandable and supportive. Fetal assessment also carries a significant ethical dimension, as it involves decision-making that affects both the mother and the unborn fetus. Interventions prompted by fetal monitoring findings, such as operative delivery or changes in labor management, must be carefully considered in light of potential risks and benefits. The nurse's role includes advocating for both patients, ensuring that care decisions are informed, respectful, and aligned with ethical principles. This dual responsibility highlights the importance of maintaining a compassionate and patient-centered approach, even in high-pressure clinical situations.

In addition to its technical and ethical aspects, fetal assessment requires a deep sense of vigilance and attentiveness. Subtle changes in fetal movement, heart rate patterns, or maternal condition may provide early of compromise, emphasizing the need for continuous observation and responsiveness. The nurse must remain alert to these, integrating them with clinical knowledge to initiate timely interventions. This ongoing process of assessment and reassessment reflects the dynamic nature of obstetric care and the critical role of the nurse in maintaining fetal well-being. Ultimately, fetal assessment is both a technical skill and a moral obligation grounded in vigilance, compassion, and respect for the unborn life. It requires the integration of advanced technology with human insight, scientific understanding with ethical awareness, and clinical precision with empathetic care. By continuously monitoring the interaction between maternal and fetal systems, interpreting findings within the broader clinical context, and responding with appropriate interventions, nurses uphold the highest standards of obstetric care. In doing so, they contribute not only to the safety and health of the fetus but also to the overall well-being and confidence of the mother, reinforcing the profound responsibility inherent in caring for two lives simultaneously.

Antenatal Testing and Predictive Value

Antenatal testing provides a critical and continuous window into the health of the fetus before the onset of labor, offering clinicians an opportunity to evaluate fetal well-being in a proactive and preventive manner rather than reacting to complications after they arise. This period of surveillance is especially significant because it allows for the early identification of potential risks that may not yet be clinically apparent through maternal symptoms alone. Through structured and systematic observation of fetal movement, heart rate variability, and placental function, clinicians are able to gather essential data that reflect the ongoing status of the intrauterine environment. These observations are not isolated measurements but components of a broader physiologic picture that helps determine whether the fetus is receiving adequate oxygen and nutrients. By identifying subtle deviations from expected patterns, healthcare providers can anticipate complications and intervene at a stage when outcomes can still be significantly improved. Tests such as the nonstress test and the biophysical profile are central to antenatal assessment, as they integrate multiple physiological signs into quantifiable and clinically meaningful indicators of fetal well-being. The nonstress test evaluates fetal heart rate patterns in response to fetal movement, providing insight into autonomic nervous system function and oxygenation status. A reactive result generally indicates adequate oxygenation and neurologic integrity, while a nonreactive result may prompt further evaluation. The biophysical profile expands this assessment by incorporating additional parameters, including fetal breathing movements, gross body movements, muscle tone, and amniotic fluid volume. Each of these components reflects a different aspect of fetal physiology, and together they create a composite score that helps guide clinical decision-making. These testing modalities demonstrate how physiologic processes can be translated into measurable indicators that support evidence-based care.

Each observation within antenatal testing—whether it is a baseline fetal heart rate, the presence of accelerations, or the measurement of amniotic fluid—represents an intricate and highly coordinated symphony of perfusion and metabolism. Adequate uteroplacental blood flow ensures the delivery of oxygen and nutrients, while efficient metabolic processes support fetal growth and development. Any disruption in this balance, such as reduced placental perfusion or impaired fetal oxygenation, can manifest as changes in these measurable parameters. Therefore, interpreting these findings requires an understanding of the underlying physiologic mechanisms that connect maternal health, placental function, and fetal response. The role of the obstetric nurse in this process is both analytical and integrative, as the nurse must interpret antenatal testing results in relation to maternal conditions such as hypertension, diabetes, or infection. These conditions can significantly influence fetal status by altering blood flow, metabolic regulation, or the intrauterine environment. For example, hypertension may reduce placental perfusion, while diabetes can affect fetal growth and metabolic balance. Recognizing that context determines meaning, the nurse must consider the entire clinical picture rather than relying solely on numerical values or isolated findings. This comprehensive approach ensures that care decisions are individualized and responsive to the specific needs of each patient.

Equally important is the ethical dimension of antenatal testing, as the results of these assessments carry significant emotional weight for patients and their families. Findings from these tests can influence critical decisions regarding the timing of delivery, the need for further interventions, or the level of monitoring required. For many patients, undergoing antenatal testing can be a source of anxiety and uncertainty, particularly when results are unclear or suggest potential complications. Sensitivity to these emotional responses is essential, and nurses play a key role in providing reassurance, clarity, and support throughout the process. Informed consent is a fundamental component of ethical care in antenatal testing, ensuring that patients understand the purpose, benefits, and potential implications of each assessment. Clear and compassionate communication helps patients feel more confident and engaged in their care, reducing fear and promoting trust in the healthcare team. The nurse's ability to explain complex procedures and in a manner that is both accurate and accessible is crucial in fostering this understanding. By addressing patient concerns and encouraging questions, nurses create an environment in which patients feel respected and supported.

Literature in midwifery and obstetric care consistently emphasizes that effective antenatal surveillance requires not only technical accuracy but also communication that empowers rather than alarms. The goal is not simply to identify potential problems but to involve patients as active participants in their care. This involves framing assessments as tools for reassurance and ongoing evaluation rather than as predictors of negative outcomes. When patients understand that testing is part of a continuous process of and support, they are more likely to engage positively with their care plan and adhere to recommended follow-up. Ultimately, the aim of antenatal testing is to promote a sense of partnership between the patient and the healthcare team. By guiding patients to understand that assessment is not a prediction of failure but an affirmation of care continuity, nurses help to shift the focus from fear to collaboration. This perspective reinforces the idea that antenatal surveillance is a proactive and supportive process designed to optimize outcomes for both mother and fetus. Through the integration of clinical expertise, ethical awareness, and compassionate communication, antenatal testing becomes not only a diagnostic tool but also a means of strengthening trust and ensuring high-quality, patient-centered care.

Nonstress and Contraction Stress Testing

The nonstress test (NST) remains a cornerstone of fetal assessment, measuring heart rate accelerations in response to movement. A reactive result implies an intact central nervous system and adequate oxygenation, while a nonreactive tracing necessitates further investigation. The contraction stress test (CST), in contrast, evaluates fetal heart rate response to uterine contractions—either spontaneous or induced—revealing placental reserve under transient hypoxia. Both methods require precise technique and interpretation. The nurse's responsibility extends beyond observation to ensuring maternal comfort, explaining the procedure, and preventing overstimulation. Continuous dialogue during testing reassures patients and enhances data reliability. Advanced obstetric manuals stress that interpretation must consider gestational age, medication effects, and sleep cycles to avoid misclassification. Each tracing embodies a narrative: the rhythm of a developing heart, the adaptation to maternal physiology, the boundary between health and distress. Accurate evaluation transforms data into decision-making that preserves fetal safety while preventing unnecessary intervention. Thus, fetal testing evolves from routine screening into an ethically conscious practice grounded in professional discernment.

Electronic Fetal Monitoring in Labor

Electronic fetal monitoring (EFM) became a defining innovation of twentieth-century obstetrics, enabling continuous surveillance of fetal heart patterns during labor. The underlying principle is to correlate heart rate variability with uterine activity to infer oxygenation. External monitoring utilizes Doppler ultrasound and tocodynamometry, while internal methods employ scalp electrodes and pressure catheters when membranes are ruptured. The obstetric nurse must master not only the technical aspects of EFM but also its interpretive complexity. Baseline rate, variability, accelerations, and decelerations together convey the story of fetal adaptation to contractions. Interpretation demands both pattern recognition and clinical reasoning, integrating maternal condition, labor stage, and medication effects. However, literature consistently reminds practitioners that technology should never replace direct patient engagement. Overreliance on monitors can distance caregivers from the human experience of birth. Ethical midwifery and nursing practice reframe EFM as an adjunct to, not a substitute for, skilled observation, touch, and empathy. The most meaningful data arise when human presence accompanies technological precision.

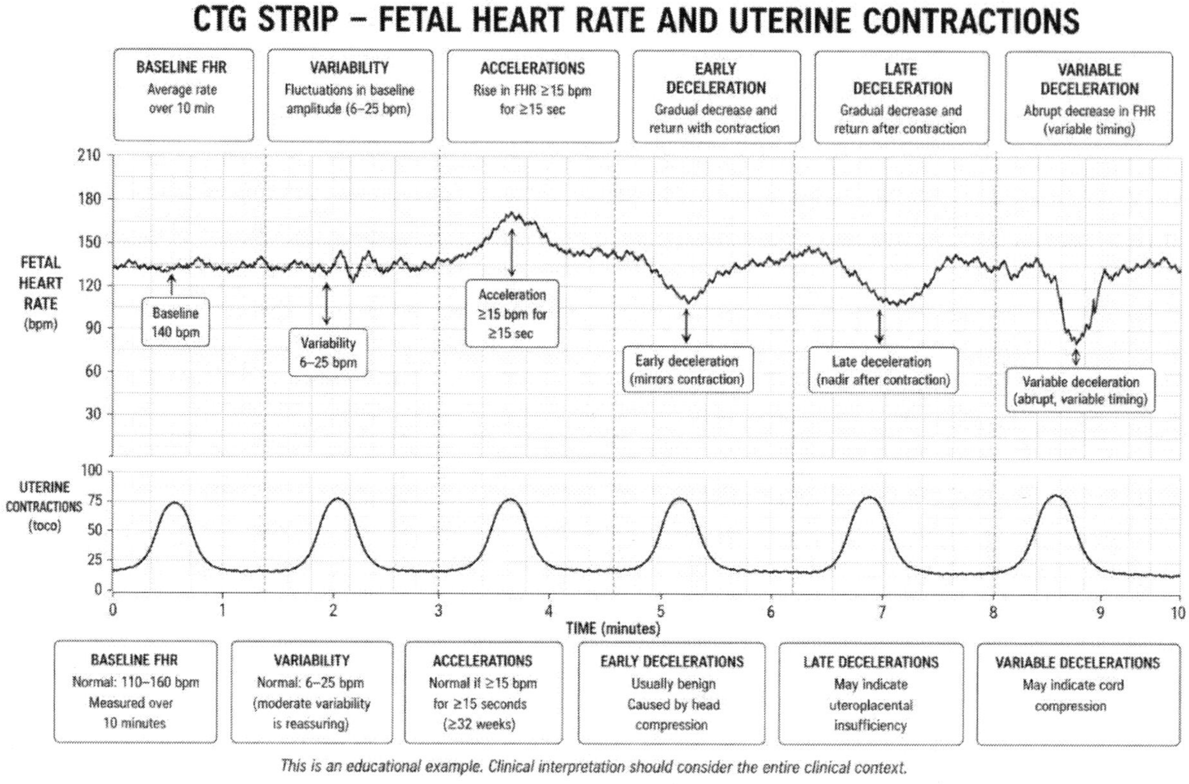

Interpreting Variability and Decelerations

Table: Fetal Heart Rate Patterns

Type	Cause	Timing	Clinical Significance
Early Decelerations	Head compression	With contractions	Benign
Late Decelerations	Uteroplacental insufficiency	After contractions	Fetal hypoxia
Variable Decelerations	Cord compression	Variable	Needs monitoring
Absent Variability	Severe distress	None	Hypoxia risk

Variability in fetal heart rate is the visual language of neurological integrity. It reflects the interplay between sympathetic and parasympathetic influences, demonstrating how the fetus responds to changing oxygen levels. Moderate variability reassures clinicians of adequate perfusion, whereas absent or minimal variability suggests compromise. Decelerations, meanwhile, offer further diagnostic clues—early decelerations mirror head compression, variable patterns imply cord involvement, and late decelerations signal uteroplacental insufficiency. The nurse's interpretive skill lies in distinguishing normal adaptive responses from warning patterns requiring escalation. Continuous correlation with contraction timing and maternal factors prevents misinterpretation. Management may involve position changes, oxygen therapy, fluid adjustment, or notifying the provider for possible delivery. Modern obstetric manuals highlight that accurate analysis stems from continuous education and reflective practice. Each tracing must be seen not as static data but as a living representation of fetal resilience. By maintaining calm vigilance and clinical reasoning, the nurse transforms observation into life-preserving action, affirming both science and compassion.

Fetal Scalp and Invasive Assessments

When noninvasive monitoring leaves uncertainty, invasive assessments provide direct insight into fetal status. Procedures such as fetal scalp blood sampling or intrauterine pressure monitoring quantify acid–base balance and contraction intensity. These methods demand advanced competency and adherence to sterile technique. The purpose is not routine diagnosis but clarification of ambiguous tracings when decisions about delivery carry high stakes. The nurse's role encompasses preparation, psychological support, and vigilant observation for complications such as infection or bleeding. Ethical guidelines emphasize that invasive testing should always rest on proportional justification—the benefits of certainty must outweigh procedural risk. Understanding the physiology behind each measurement allows nurses to interpret results accurately and advocate for patient-centered choices. In high-risk scenarios, invasive assessment can distinguish reversible hypoxia from irreversible compromise, guiding timely intervention. Such precision underscores the partnership between clinical science and professional ethics, where every act of assessment seeks the balance between knowledge and safety.

Non-Electronic and Adjunctive Techniques

Even in the era of advanced monitoring, fundamental methods like auscultation, palpation, and maternal perception of movement retain enduring value. These low-technology assessments rely on attentive listening and human connection. Intermittent auscultation, when performed skillfully, provides reliable information on baseline heart rate and response to contractions while preserving mobility and privacy. Palpation of contractions enables evaluation of frequency, intensity, and resting tone without mechanical assistance. Maternal awareness of fetal movement offers another dimension of assessment, empowering individuals to participate actively in their own surveillance. Educational materials in modern midwifery reaffirm that these techniques maintain sensitivity and respect for physiologic birth while safeguarding safety. Nurses who blend manual skills with modern tools preserve a holistic perspective. The essence of obstetric care lies not only in precision but in presence—the assurance that even amid technology, the nurse's attentive senses remain the most responsive instruments in protecting life.

Fetal Acid-Base and Oxygenation Assessment

Understanding fetal oxygenation extends beyond heart rate interpretation to biochemical analysis of acid–base status. During stress, anaerobic metabolism produces lactic acid, lowering pH and signaling hypoxia. Sampling from cord blood or scalp capillaries provides quantitative confirmation of fetal reserve. Such evaluation transforms subjective tracing interpretation into measurable data. However, interpretation demands careful contextualization: transient acidemia may occur with vigorous labor yet resolve spontaneously. The obstetric nurse's task is to integrate laboratory findings with clinical presentation, ensuring that interventions remain proportionate. Fluid resuscitation, oxygen supplementation, or expedited delivery may be indicated depending on the pattern. Current obstetric literature underscores that acid–base analysis bridges physiology and ethics—each value represents more than chemistry; it signifies a decision point that can alter two lives simultaneously. Precision, patience, and interdisciplinary dialogue define the responsible use of biochemical fetal assessment within modern perinatal care.

Communication, Ethics, and Professional Accountability

Fetal monitoring produces vast streams of data, but its true value depends on accurate interpretation, timely communication, and ethical integrity. Documentation of patterns, interventions, and provider notifications forms the legal and moral backbone of intrapartum nursing. Misinterpretation or delayed escalation can have lifelong consequences. Ethical frameworks within professional nursing emphasize beneficence, nonmaleficence, and respect for autonomy as guiding principles in every decision. Nurses must balance clinical judgment with transparency, ensuring that patients understand both the purpose and limits of monitoring. Effective teamwork—structured hand-offs, interdisciplinary debriefs, and situational awareness—strengthens safety. The professional's inner commitment to truth and accountability transforms technical monitoring into moral practice. Every tracing, every report, and every decision must reflect not only competence but conscience. Within the heartbeat's rhythm lies the essence of nursing ethics: to observe with skill, to act with courage, and to speak with integrity for those yet unable to speak for themselves.

The Role of the Nurse in Continuous Fetal Observation

The obstetric nurse serves as both scientist and sentinel in the ongoing process of fetal observation. Beyond operating monitoring equipment, the nurse interprets physiologic data through the lens of experience and empathy. Continuous assessment demands an alert mind that can discern patterns amid the noise of contractions, movement, and maternal variables. The nurse must maintain uninterrupted attention to the evolving clinical picture, correlating findings with interventions and patient responses. Critical thinking guides moment-to-moment decisions, such as adjusting maternal position or recommending further evaluation. Communication with the multidisciplinary team ensures that emerging concerns are addressed collaboratively and without delay. Within this dynamic setting, the nurse also fulfills an emotional role, translating complex information into reassurance for the patient and family. The ethical dimension of observation lies in advocacy—the responsibility to speak when subtle warning signs appear. Thus, the nurse's sustained vigilance transforms technical monitoring into compassionate guardianship of maternal and fetal life.

Cultural and Psychosocial Dimensions of Fetal Monitoring

Fetal assessment does not occur in a vacuum of technology but within the cultural and emotional landscape of each birthing family. Beliefs about childbirth, privacy, and medical intervention influence how patients perceive monitoring procedures. Some may welcome continuous surveillance as safety assurance, while others experience it as invasive or disempowering. The nurse's role is to navigate these sensitivities with cultural humility and individualized explanation. Recognizing the patient's values allows for negotiation of care that honors autonomy without compromising safety. Psychosocial factors such as anxiety, previous trauma, or language barriers can alter physiological responses, even affecting heart rate patterns. Supportive communication, respect for personal boundaries, and inclusion of family in the discussion foster trust. Midwifery and ethics literature alike emphasize that true assessment begins with listening—both to the fetal heart and to the mother's voice. When culture and compassion align, fetal surveillance becomes not merely a test but a shared journey toward a safe and dignified birth.

Documentation and Legal Accountability in Fetal Assessment

Accurate documentation forms the bridge between observation and accountability in obstetric nursing. Every tracing, interpretation, and intervention must be recorded with precision, reflecting real-time events and rationale. Documentation provides continuity of care, allowing incoming staff and providers to understand clinical progression and prior responses. In the event of adverse outcomes, these records become the objective evidence of professional diligence. Legal and ethical frameworks highlight that incomplete or retrospective charting undermines both patient safety and professional credibility. The nurse's notes should capture not only numerical data but the clinical reasoning that guided decisions. When uncertainty arises, collaboration and documentation of consultation preserve transparency. Contemporary nursing ethics emphasize that thorough recording is an act of advocacy—it ensures the patient's story is told accurately and protects both nurse and patient from misrepresentation. In the realm of fetal assessment, documentation is more than administrative duty; it is the written heartbeat of accountability.

Integration of Technology and Human Judgment

Modern obstetric care stands at the convergence of digital precision and human intuition. Sophisticated monitoring systems now provide real-time analytics, remote tracing review, and computerized alerts. Yet, technology alone cannot replace the interpretive wisdom of the experienced clinician. Machines record patterns; humans assign meaning. The challenge lies in harmonizing technological efficiency with human empathy. Overreliance on automated interpretation risks complacency, while rejection of innovation forfeits valuable insight. The nurse's task is to integrate both—using data as an extension of critical thought rather than its replacement. Education and ongoing simulation training strengthen this balance, enabling nurses to respond swiftly without surrendering reflection. Literature on ethics in contemporary nursing underscores that technology should amplify, not diminish, compassion. When applied judiciously, electronic monitoring becomes a partner in caregiving, translating invisible physiologic whispers into actionable knowledge. True mastery lies in seeing beyond the screen—to recognize that every waveform reflects a living bond between two interdependent hearts.

Chapter 3: Labor and Birth

The Physiology of Labor

Labor represents one of the most complex and finely coordinated physiological transformations in human biology, marked by the synchronized and interdependent efforts of the uterus, cervix, endocrine system, and fetal signaling mechanisms. This process is not abrupt but develops gradually through a series of preparatory changes that begin well before the onset of clinically recognized labor. These preparatory phases involve cervical ripening, increased uterine sensitivity, and hormonal priming, all of which create the conditions necessary for effective labor. The onset of true labor arises from a delicate and precisely regulated biochemical dialogue in which progesterone withdrawal, oxytocin receptor upregulation, and prostaglandin release converge to initiate rhythmic and increasingly effective uterine contractions. This transition reflects a shift from uterine quiescence to active contractility, demonstrating the remarkable adaptability of the maternal body in preparing for childbirth. These uterine contractions play a central role in the labor process, progressively effacing and dilating the cervix while simultaneously promoting the descent of the presenting fetal part through the birth canal. Effacement involves the thinning and shortening of the cervical tissue, while dilation refers to the gradual opening of the cervical os, both of which are essential for allowing the passage of the fetus. The force generated by uterine contractions is transmitted downward, guiding the fetus into alignment with the maternal pelvis. This mechanical process is closely linked with biochemical changes, as the release of prostaglandins further enhances cervical softening and uterine activity. The coordination of these events ensures that labor progresses in an organized and efficient manner, minimizing trauma and optimizing outcomes for both mother and fetus.

At the cellular level, myometrial cells play a critical role in facilitating effective uterine contractions. These cells communicate through specialized structures known as gap junctions, which allow electrical impulses to pass rapidly from one cell to another. This communication enables the uterus to function as a single, unified organ rather than as a collection of individual muscle fibers. As labor approaches, the number of gap junctions increases significantly, enhancing the synchronization of contractions and ensuring that they occur in a coordinated and powerful manner. This transformation of the uterus into a single functional unit is essential for generating the force required to achieve cervical dilation and fetal descent. Hormonal interplay further intensifies and regulates the labor process, creating a complex network of feedback mechanisms that sustain and amplify uterine activity. Oxytocin, released from the posterior pituitary gland, plays a central role in this process by stimulating uterine contractions and promoting the release of additional prostaglandins from the decidua and fetal membranes. This creates a positive feedback loop in which contractions stimulate further oxytocin release, leading to progressively stronger and more frequent contractions. At the same time, the reduction in progesterone's inhibitory effects allows estrogen to enhance uterine sensitivity, further facilitating contractility. This intricate hormonal balance ensures that labor progresses in a controlled yet effective manner.

In addition to its mechanical and hormonal components, labor also involves significant neurophysiological adaptations that support maternal coping and participation in the birth process. The release of endorphins, which are natural pain-relieving substances produced by the body, helps the mother manage the discomfort associated with contractions and promotes a sense of focus and resilience. As labor advances, particularly during the second stage, surges in catecholamines such as epinephrine and norepinephrine enhance alertness and provide the needed for effective pushing efforts. These physiologic responses demonstrate how the body prepares not only for the physical demands of labor but also for the and emotional challenges that accompany childbirth. Clinically, recognition and understanding of this complex physiology underpin safe and effective labor management. Healthcare providers, particularly nurses, must be able to distinguish between normal labor progression and signs of dysfunction or complication. This requires careful assessment of contraction patterns, cervical changes, fetal response, and maternal condition. Interventions, when necessary, should be guided by an understanding of the underlying physiologic processes, ensuring that they support rather than disrupt the natural progression of labor. For example, the use of oxytocin for labor augmentation must be carefully titrated to enhance contractions without causing uterine hyperstimulation or fetal distress.

Understanding labor as a balance between biology and adaptation ensures that clinical care remains supportive of natural mechanisms rather than unnecessarily invasive. Each stage of labor reflects a carefully orchestrated sequence of events that has evolved to optimize the process of birth. Respecting this process involves allowing time for physiologic changes to occur while remaining prepared to intervene when deviations from normal patterns threaten maternal or fetal well-being. This balanced approach promotes safer outcomes and enhances the overall birth experience. Ultimately, each contraction represents more than a mechanical force; it reflects the culmination of evolutionary design and physiologic coordination. Labor is an orchestrated effort involving tissue, hormones, neural pathways, and maternal will, all working together toward the creation of new life. The integration of these elements highlights the remarkable complexity and resilience of the human body, as well as the critical role of skilled clinical care in supporting this transformative process.

The Onset and Stages of Labor

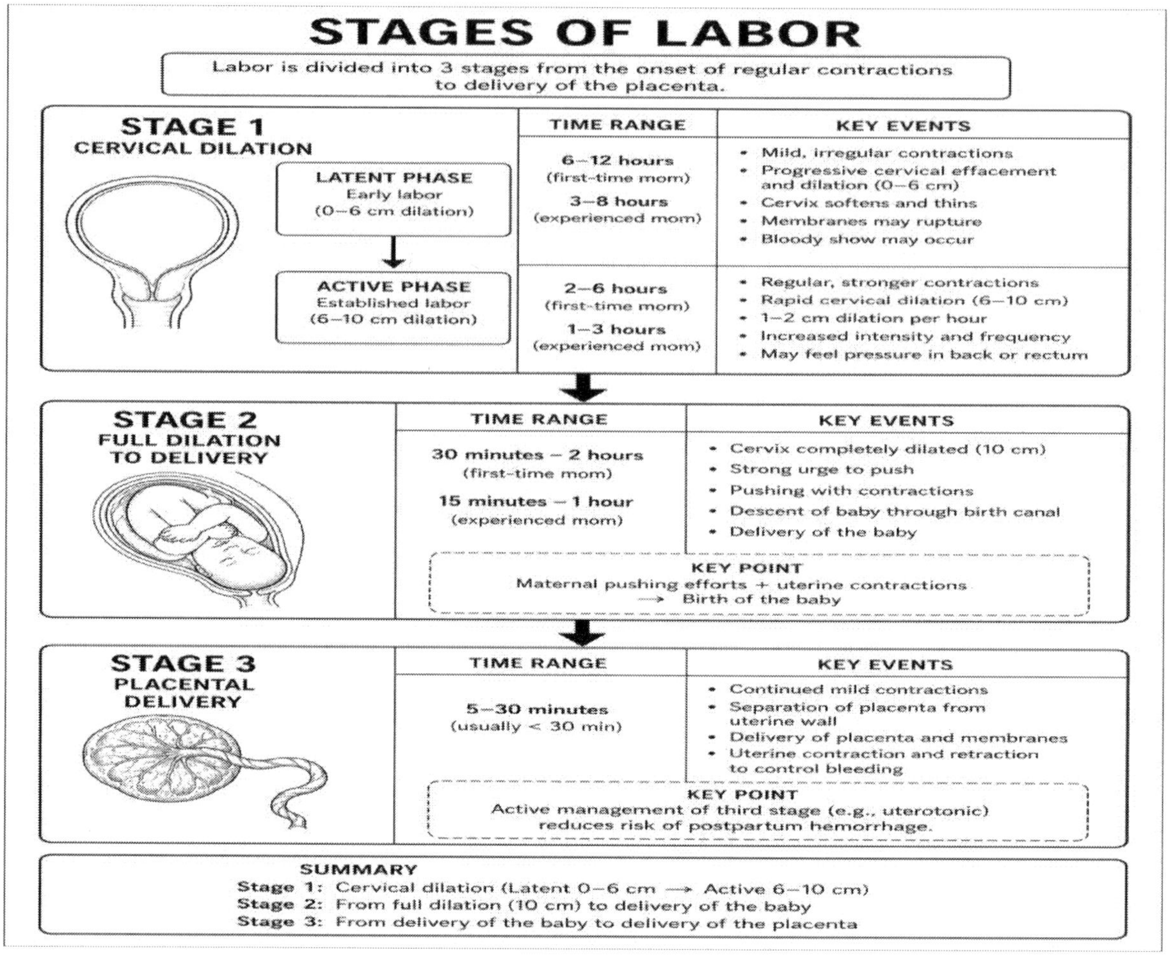

The onset of labor is identified by regular, painful contractions that lead to progressive cervical dilation and effacement. It is traditionally divided into three stages: dilation, expulsion, and placental delivery. The first stage spans the latent and active phases, characterized by cervical ripening and then rapid dilation beyond six centimeters. The second stage commences with full dilation and culminates in the birth of the baby, a phase that blends involuntary uterine power with maternal bearing-down efforts. The third stage begins after delivery and concludes with placental separation. Each stage carries distinct physiological and emotional demands. The midwife's awareness of these transitions allows anticipatory care that reduces anxiety and preserves energy. From a biological perspective, the timing of onset varies with maternal readiness, fetal maturity, and uterine sensitivity. This unpredictability demands that nurses remain both vigilant and flexible, supporting labor's innate variability while identifying deviations that require medical collaboration. Thus, understanding stages of labor combines precision with patience—a balance central to obstetric artistry.

Cervical Effacement and Dilation

Effacement and dilation are the visible outcomes of complex cervical remodeling under the influence of mechanical forces and biochemical mediators. Collagen fibers within the cervix undergo enzymatic softening, increasing elasticity while reducing structural rigidity. Prostaglandins and estrogen heighten tissue responsiveness, allowing cervical fibers to stretch as the presenting part descends. The process begins with effacement—the thinning of the cervix—followed by dilation, the measurable widening of the cervical canal. Clinically, these changes are assessed through sterile vaginal examination, though contemporary guidance stresses minimal intrusion to prevent infection and preserve privacy. The rate of dilation varies, influenced by parity, fetal position, and contraction efficiency. Nurses translate these findings into ongoing evaluations of progress, providing reassurance that slow dilation can still signify normal physiology. The cervix, once a barrier, transforms into a gateway through which life emerges. Observing this transition with respect and restraint exemplifies the professionalism and empathy foundational to obstetric nursing.

Maternal Adaptations During Labor

Labor imposes profound and multifaceted physiological adjustments that test the limits of human endurance, requiring the coordinated effort of multiple organ systems to sustain both maternal function and fetal well-being. These adjustments begin early in labor and intensify as contractions become more frequent and forceful, placing increasing demands on cardiovascular, respiratory, endocrine, and metabolic systems. The body responds to these demands through adaptive mechanisms that are both immediate and sustained, ensuring that adequate oxygen, energy, and perfusion are maintained throughout the labor process. Rather than representing dysfunction, these changes reflect the body's capacity to adapt to one of the most physically demanding events in human experience. Cardiovascular output may increase significantly during labor, in some cases nearly doubling from baseline levels, as the heart works more efficiently to redistribute blood flow to essential areas, particularly the uterus and placenta. Each uterine contraction temporarily reduces blood flow to the placenta, creating intermittent periods of decreased fetal oxygenation that must be compensated for by increased maternal cardiac output between contractions. This cyclical pattern requires precise regulation to ensure that both maternal tissues and the fetus receive adequate perfusion. Blood pressure may fluctuate in response to pain, anxiety, and contraction intensity, further emphasizing the need for continuous monitoring. These cardiovascular adjustments illustrate how the maternal body prioritizes uterine activity while maintaining systemic stability.

Respiratory changes also play a critical role in supporting the increased metabolic demands of labor. As contractions intensify, respiratory rates rise, often accompanied by deeper breathing patterns as the body attempts to meet heightened oxygen requirements. Hyperventilation may occur, particularly in response to pain or anxiety, leading to a state of mild respiratory alkalosis characterized by decreased carbon dioxide levels in the blood. While this condition is generally well tolerated, it may produce symptoms such as dizziness, tingling, or lightheadedness, requiring reassurance and guidance in controlled breathing techniques. Effective respiratory adaptation ensures that oxygen delivery remains sufficient for both maternal tissues and fetal needs during the stress of labor. Endocrine changes further enhance the body's ability to sustain labor by increasing sensitivity to key hormones such as oxytocin and catecholamines. Oxytocin facilitates uterine contractions, strengthening their intensity and coordination, while catecholamines influence both cardiovascular responses and pain perception. The interplay of these hormones creates a dynamic environment in which uterine activity is amplified and maternal alertness is heightened, particularly in the later stages of labor. At the same time, endorphins are released, providing a natural mechanism for pain relief and contributing to the mother's ability to cope with the physical demands of labor. This complex hormonal balance demonstrates how the body integrates multiple systems to support both function and endurance.

Fluid shifts and electrolyte balance represent another critical aspect of physiologic adaptation during labor, particularly in cases of prolonged or intense labor. Sweating, increased expenditure, and limited oral intake can lead to dehydration and electrolyte imbalances if not carefully managed. Intravenous fluids or oral hydration may be necessary to maintain adequate circulating volume and prevent complications such as hypotension or fatigue. Continuous observation of fluid status, including urine output and signs of dehydration, is essential to ensure that the body's internal environment remains stable throughout the labor process. Emotional adaptation parallels these physical changes, creating a complex and evolving psychological landscape in which anxiety, excitement, anticipation, and exhaustion coexist in a fluid continuum. The uncertainty of labor progression, combined with the intensity of physical sensations, can heighten emotional responses and influence coping ability. The presence of supportive care providers plays a crucial role in shaping this experience, as reassurance, encouragement, and clear communication can significantly reduce anxiety and enhance confidence. Emotional well-being is closely linked to physiologic stability, as stress and fear may increase catecholamine levels, potentially interfering with effective uterine contractions.

The midwife's role extends beyond the monitoring of vital signs and clinical parameters to include the recognition of subtle signs of fatigue, distress, or emotional overwhelm. Observing changes in behavior, levels, or coping patterns allows for early intervention that can prevent further deterioration. Simple measures such as repositioning, providing hydration, offering comfort measures, and encouraging rest between contractions can have a profound impact on the patient's ability to sustain labor. These interventions support both physical endurance and emotional resilience, reinforcing the importance of holistic care. Encouragement and continuous support are essential components of maintaining morale during labor, as they help the patient remain engaged and motivated despite increasing fatigue. Verbal reassurance, presence, and attentive care contribute to a sense of safety and trust, which in turn facilitates more effective coping strategies. Positioning interventions, such as upright or lateral positions, can improve comfort, enhance uterine efficiency, and promote fetal descent, demonstrating how simple adjustments can influence physiologic outcomes.

Through these extensive adjustments, the laboring body demonstrates remarkable resilience and adaptability, transforming physiologic stress into a purposeful and productive process. What might otherwise be perceived as strain or imbalance becomes a coordinated effort directed toward the goal of childbirth. This transformation underscores the importance of understanding labor not as a pathological state but as a normal physiologic event that requires support rather than correction. Physiological stress becomes purposeful rather than pathological when guided by informed and compassionate care, a principle deeply embedded in midwifery tradition and consistently reinforced by evidence-based obstetric practice. By integrating clinical knowledge with empathetic support, healthcare providers can ensure that the laboring individual is not only physically supported but also emotionally empowered. This approach recognizes that successful labor outcomes depend not only on physiologic processes but also on the quality of care, communication, and human connection provided throughout the experience.

Fetal Descent and Mechanisms of Labor

The passage of the fetus through the birth canal follows a predictable sequence of movements known as the mechanisms of labor: engagement, descent, flexion, internal rotation, extension, restitution, and expulsion. Each motion aligns the fetal head optimally within the maternal pelvis, minimizing resistance. Pelvic architecture and fetal lie influence this choreography; even minor deviations can alter progression.

Nurses and midwives are trained to interpret these mechanisms not merely as anatomical descriptions but as living processes unfolding before them. Palpation, observation of contraction patterns, and assessment of presenting part descent allow real-time evaluation of progress. Encouraging upright positioning and mobility enhances pelvic dimensions and facilitates descent. These biomechanical insights underscore the partnership between maternal effort and fetal cooperation. Birth thus emerges not as a passive event but as an active collaboration between two bodies aligned in purpose and effort, reflecting the intricate intelligence of human physiology.

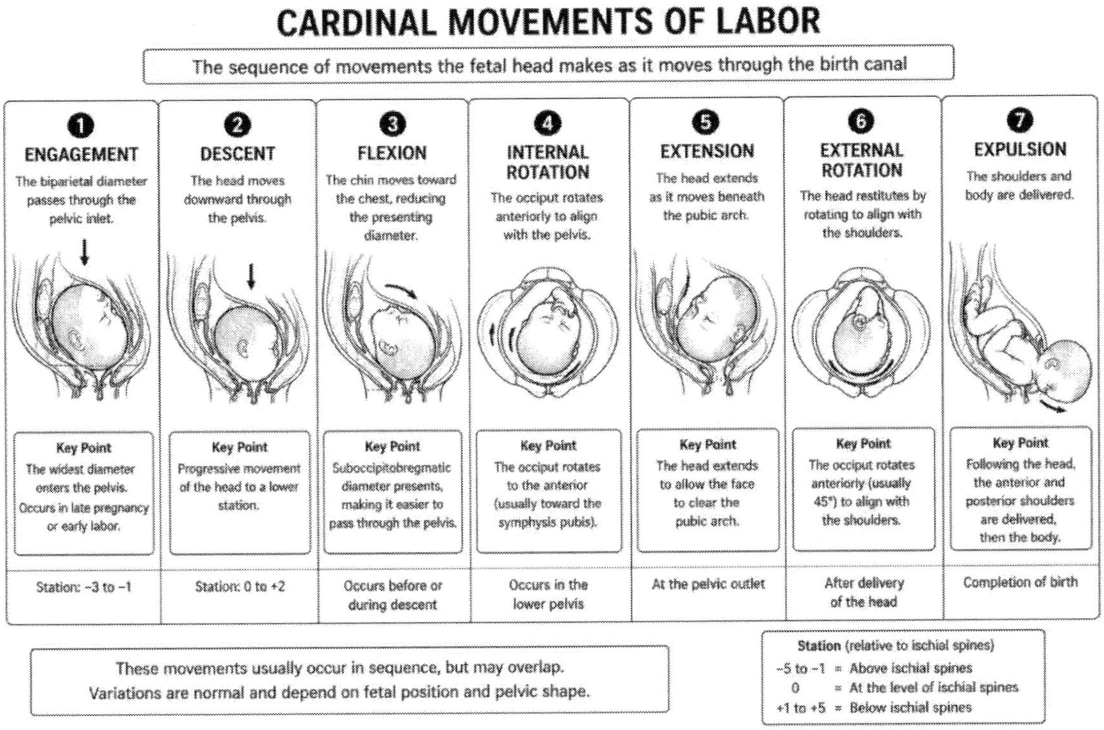

Maternal Pain and Physiological Coping

Pain during labor is both a deeply physical and profoundly existential experience, shaped not only by the physiologic processes of childbirth but also by emotional, psychological, and cultural influences. It arises primarily from uterine contractions, cervical dilation, and the progressive descent of the fetus, yet its perception varies widely among individuals depending on prior experiences, expectations, and support systems. The source of discomfort lies in the activation of visceral and somatic afferent pathways, which transmit pain signals generated by uterine ischemia during contractions and by stretching of the cervix, vagina, and perineum as labor advances. These physiologic mechanisms explain the intensity and evolving nature of labor pain, which typically begins as diffuse, cramping discomfort and becomes more localized and intense as the fetus descends and tissues stretch.

Despite its intensity, labor pain also carries significant meaning, extending beyond physical sensation to encompass emotional and symbolic dimensions. For many individuals, pain signifies progress, vitality, and the anticipation of birth, transforming it from a purely negative experience into one that is purposeful and meaningful. This dual nature of pain—as both challenge and indicator of advancement—highlights the importance of understanding labor not only in physiologic terms but also within the broader context of human experience. Recognizing this meaning allows healthcare providers to support patients in reframing pain as a component of the birth process rather than solely as suffering. Physiologic coping mechanisms play a critical role in modulating the perception of pain and supporting the laboring individual's ability to endure contractions. The release of endorphins, the body's natural analgesics, increases as labor progresses, helping to reduce pain intensity and promote a sense of focus and resilience. Rhythmic breathing techniques further enhance coping by improving oxygenation, reducing muscle tension, and providing a sense of control over the body's responses. These natural strategies demonstrate the body's inherent capacity to adapt to the demands of labor and to mitigate discomfort through internal regulatory processes.

The presence of supportive care significantly influences the experience of pain, as emotional reassurance and continuous companionship can reduce anxiety and decrease the release of catecholamines associated with stress. Elevated catecholamine levels may interfere with effective uterine contractions and reduce uterine perfusion, potentially prolonging labor and increasing discomfort. By providing calm, consistent support and clear communication, nurses and other caregivers help create an environment that promotes relaxation and physiologic efficiency. This supportive presence not only alleviates emotional distress but also contributes to improved clinical outcomes. The nurse's role in pain management extends beyond observation to active guidance in techniques that harmonize the mind and body. Interventions such as relaxation exercises, hydrotherapy, massage, and movement encourage comfort and enhance the body's natural coping mechanisms. Position changes, for example, can reduce pressure, improve fetal alignment, and facilitate labor progression, while warm water immersion may provide soothing relief and reduce muscle tension. These nonpharmacologic approaches emphasize the importance of individualized care, allowing patients to explore methods that align with their preferences and needs.

Modern perspectives on labor pain management emphasize the principle of choice, recognizing that each patient's experience and tolerance of pain are unique. Both pharmacologic and nonpharmacologic strategies are considered valid and valuable, and decisions regarding their use should be guided by patient preference, clinical indications, and ongoing assessment. Pharmacologic options, such as regional anesthesia or systemic analgesics, provide effective pain relief when needed, while nonpharmacologic methods offer alternatives that support physiologic processes and personal autonomy. This flexible approach ensures that care remains patient-centered and responsive to changing circumstances during labor. Importantly, pain management in labor transcends the simple goal of analgesia, reflecting a broader ethical commitment to preserving dignity, autonomy, and a sense of control. The manner in which pain is addressed can significantly influence the overall birth experience, shaping memories and perceptions long after delivery. Respecting patient choices, providing informed consent, and maintaining open communication are essential components of ethical care that honor the individual's and participation in decision-making.

To understand pain in labor is to recognize and respect the strength and resilience of the laboring individual. Each contraction represents not only a physiologic effort but also a moment of endurance and determination, bringing the patient closer to the culmination of the birth process. By supporting patients through this experience with knowledge, compassion, and respect, healthcare providers help ensure that pain becomes a meaningful and manageable aspect of labor rather than an overwhelming burden. Ultimately, effective pain management transforms the experience of labor from one of uncontrolled suffering into one of empowered participation. Through a combination of physiologic understanding, supportive care, and individualized intervention, nurses play a pivotal role in helping patients navigate the challenges of labor. In doing so, they uphold the principle that each contraction is not merely a source of discomfort but a purposeful step toward the creation of new life, reinforcing the idea that pain, when understood and supported, can become a pathway to strength and triumph.

Fetal Monitoring During Labor

Fetal monitoring during labor provides continuous insight into the physiologic dialogue between mother and fetus. Through external cardiotocography or intermittent auscultation, clinicians observe heart rate patterns that mirror oxygenation and neurological integrity. Interpretation focuses on baseline rate, variability, accelerations, and decelerations. Internal monitoring, when indicated, enhances precision but carries risks of infection or injury. Evidence supports individualized monitoring strategies: low-risk labors often benefit from intermittent auscultation, while high-risk situations justify continuous surveillance. The nurse's interpretive skill ensures that abnormalities are recognized promptly and interventions—such as repositioning or oxygen therapy—are executed effectively. Importantly, monitoring should complement, not dominate, the birthing experience. Ethical care demands that technology serves the woman, not the reverse. Within the rhythmic tracing of a fetal heart lies a narrative of endurance, adaptation, and hope—the silent testament of life preparing to emerge.

Induction and Augmentation of Labor

Induction and augmentation represent deliberate interventions designed to initiate or enhance uterine contractions when natural labor fails to progress or when maternal or fetal conditions necessitate delivery. The process must always balance medical necessity with physiological respect. Oxytocin infusion, prostaglandin administration, and membrane sweeping are among the primary methods, each requiring meticulous monitoring of contraction patterns and fetal well-being. Induction without clear indication risks hyperstimulation, fetal distress, or operative delivery; therefore, careful patient selection and informed consent are essential. The nurse plays a central role in titrating medications, assessing uterine response, and maintaining open communication with the laboring woman. Augmentation of spontaneous labor, when performed judiciously, can restore normal rhythm and prevent exhaustion. Yet evidence consistently affirms that patience—allowing the body's hormonal orchestration to unfold—is often the safest approach. In essence, induction and augmentation reveal the art of obstetric timing: knowing when to intervene and when to wait, always guided by the principle of safety above speed.

Obstetric and Perioperative Procedures

Modern obstetrics bridges natural and surgical disciplines, demanding that nurses possess proficiency across both. Procedures such as artificial rupture of membranes, epidural anesthesia placement, episiotomy, and cesarean birth require collaboration and precision. Each intervention carries physiological consequences that must be understood and anticipated. For example, rupture of membranes alters fetal cushioning and infection risk, while regional anesthesia affects maternal hemodynamics and mobility. The perioperative nurse safeguards sterile technique, prepares equipment, and provides emotional grounding during transitions from labor to surgery. In cesarean delivery, coordinated teamwork ensures rapid neonatal assessment and uterine repair under aseptic conditions. Recovery care involves vigilant monitoring for hemorrhage, pain control, and emotional adjustment. The nurse's presence offers continuity across procedural boundaries, reminding every patient that even within high-technology environments, compassionate touch remains the most vital instrument. Obstetric procedures exemplify the fusion of science and empathy—each incision and intervention guided by purpose, precision, and respect.

Management of Labor Complications

Complications during labor can arise suddenly, transforming routine progress into urgent intervention. Conditions such as shoulder dystocia, cord prolapse, uterine rupture, and amniotic fluid embolism challenge even experienced teams. Early recognition through skilled observation remains the cornerstone of safety. The nurse, often first to detect subtle warning signs, must act decisively while maintaining calm communication. Position changes, relief of cord pressure, and activation of emergency protocols are executed with disciplined speed. Manuals on obstetric emergencies emphasize that success depends not solely on knowledge but on rehearsal—team drills and role clarity reduce delay and confusion. Emotional management of the patient and family is equally critical, as crises magnify fear. Effective communication transforms chaos into coordinated response. Through training and composure, nurses embody the resilience required in obstetric emergencies, demonstrating that competence under pressure is not instinct but cultivated professionalism grounded in preparation and compassion.

Pain Relief and Anesthetic Considerations

Pain relief in labor represents a spectrum ranging from nonpharmacologic support to regional or systemic analgesia. Choice depends on patient preference, clinical condition, and stage of labor. Epidural analgesia remains the most effective method for severe pain but requires continuous assessment for hypotension and fetal response. Opioids offer temporary relief but may influence neonatal respiration. Nonpharmacologic methods—breathing, hydrotherapy, massage, and hypnosis—enhance relaxation without pharmacologic side effects. The nurse's role involves educating patients about options, supporting decision-making, and monitoring for complications. Ethical frameworks highlight autonomy and informed consent as central to pain management. Comfort, safety, and dignity coexist when interventions align with patient values. Effective analgesia not only relieves pain but preserves psychological integrity, transforming the birthing process into an experience of controlled strength. Thus, anesthesia in labor is more than a medical service; it is a dialogue between biology and empathy, grounded in trust and vigilance.

Teamwork and Communication in the Birth Environment

Safe childbirth depends as much on human interaction as on technical proficiency. Teamwork in labor units involves synchronization among nurses, midwives, physicians, anesthetists, and neonatologists. Communication errors are a leading cause of preventable obstetric harm; therefore, structured communication tools such as SBAR (Situation, Background, Assessment, Recommendation) are essential. The nurse often serves as the communication anchor—coordinating updates, relaying concerns, and ensuring every team member shares the same mental model. Respectful collaboration reduces hierarchy-induced hesitation and fosters timely escalation. Emotional intelligence, empathy, and cultural awareness enhance teamwork, particularly during high-stress scenarios. Reflective debriefings after complex births reinforce learning and psychological safety. Literature on obstetric emergencies emphasizes that human factors, not knowledge deficits, often determine outcomes. When teams listen as well as they act, the labor room becomes an ecosystem of competence and compassion, where every professional voice contributes to the symphony of safe birth.

Family-Centered Support and Cultural Sensitivity

Labor and birth occur within a cultural and emotional context that defines meaning as much as outcome. Family-centered care recognizes the birthing individual as part of a relational unit whose needs extend beyond the physical. Cultural beliefs shape preferences regarding pain expression, birth position, and decision-making roles. Sensitivity to these values transforms care from procedural to personal. The nurse's role includes facilitating inclusion, encouraging partner participation, and ensuring privacy and respect. Effective communication overcomes barriers of language or custom, turning diversity into strength. In some cultures, the presence of extended family or specific rituals provides comfort; in others, solitude and modesty are paramount. By adapting practice without compromising safety, nurses honor individuality within a universal experience. Cultural competence is therefore not mere courtesy but an ethical responsibility—acknowledging that birth is at once biological, spiritual, and deeply human.

Transition to Postpartum Care

The moments following delivery represent both culmination and beginning. As the placenta separates and the uterus contracts, attention shifts from delivery to stabilization. Monitoring for hemorrhage, uterine tone, and vital signs ensures physiological safety, while emotional support fosters psychological transition. Immediate skin-to-skin contact promotes thermoregulation, bonding, and initiation of breastfeeding. The nurse assesses perineal integrity, manages pain, and provides reassurance as the mother adjusts to profound physical and hormonal change. The third stage's management—whether physiological or active—requires vigilance for retained tissue or atony. Concurrently, family engagement reinforces shared joy and confidence in newborn care. Transition to postpartum recovery closes the cycle of labor but opens the journey of parenting. Within this moment, the nurse's calm presence bridges exhaustion and triumph, guiding the family through their first steps in a new chapter of life that began with labor's enduring rhythm and ends in the quiet heartbeat of belonging.

Chapter 4: Recovery, Postpartum, and Newborn Care

The Physiology of Postpartum Recovery

Table: Postpartum Changes

System	Normal Change	Time Frame	Clinical Concern
Uterus	Involution	~6 weeks	Subinvolution
Lochia	Rubra → Serosa → Alba	Up to 6 weeks	Hemorrhage
Breasts	Milk production	2–3 days	Mastitis
Cardiovascular	↑ CO then normal	~2 weeks	Thromboembolism

The postpartum period, often called the fourth stage of labor, marks a complex transition where the mother's body gradually returns to its nonpregnant state while adapting to the demands of newborn care. The uterus begins involution through sustained myometrial contractions, reducing its size and minimizing bleeding. Hormonal shifts occur rapidly—estrogen and progesterone levels fall, while prolactin and oxytocin rise, influencing lactation and emotional bonding. Circulatory volume normalizes, renal function accelerates diuresis, and metabolic rates decline. Despite these physiologic recalibrations, the body remains vulnerable to infection and hemorrhage, demanding careful observation. Nurses monitor vital signs, uterine tone, lochia, and perineal integrity to detect early warning signs of complications. Emotional changes accompany physical recovery, from elation to fatigue or transient mood shifts. The nurse's role encompasses reassurance, rest facilitation, and education about expected changes. Recognizing that recovery involves both physical healing and psychological integration ensures a holistic approach. The postpartum body, though weakened by exertion, possesses remarkable resilience—each contraction, breath, and tear marking progress toward renewed equilibrium.

Uterine Involution and Hemodynamic Stability

Uterine involution symbolizes the restoration of reproductive anatomy after childbirth. Immediately post-delivery, the uterus weighs about one kilogram; within six weeks, it contracts to approximately 60 grams. This transformation depends on sustained oxytocin-mediated contractions, which compress uterine vessels and prevent hemorrhage. The nurse palpates fundal position and firmness regularly, ensuring it descends predictably toward the pelvis. A boggy uterus or excessive bleeding demands prompt intervention through massage, bladder emptying, or pharmacologic agents such as oxytocin or misoprostol. Hemodynamic stability remains a concurrent priority, as blood loss during delivery can precipitate hypovolemia. Monitoring heart rate, blood pressure, and hematocrit trends provides objective evaluation. Adequate hydration and iron supplementation promote recovery. The postpartum nurse's vigilance often determines early identification of atony or concealed bleeding, preventing severe morbidity. Beyond technique lies attentiveness—the ability to read subtle cues of pallor, anxiety, or fatigue that precede measurable decline. Uterine involution thus represents not merely anatomy but the disciplined choreography of nursing observation safeguarding maternal life.

Perineal Integrity and Wound Healing

Perineal recovery after vaginal birth involves complex tissue repair influenced by vascular supply, cleanliness, and mobility. First- and second-degree lacerations usually heal without complication, while deeper tears or episiotomy require careful suturing and hygiene maintenance. Pain, edema, and bruising are expected but should diminish progressively. The nurse's responsibilities include inspecting for signs of hematoma, infection, or wound separation while respecting privacy and cultural modesty. Cold compresses, sitz baths, and analgesia support comfort. Encouraging pelvic floor exercises restores muscle tone and enhances circulation, promoting healing. Education about hygiene, avoidance of strain, and gradual resumption of activity empowers self-care. Evidence-based guidelines highlight that empathy and communication are as essential as clinical skill in perineal management. For many women, discomfort carries emotional sensitivity linked to body image and intimacy. By fostering dignity and reassurance, nurses transform perineal care from a technical task into an act of restorative respect—reaffirming comfort, safety, and confidence in the early days of motherhood.

Lactation Physiology and Breast Care

Lactation is a hormonally driven process rooted in maternal adaptation and emotional connection. The decline in estrogen and progesterone after delivery releases prolactin from pituitary inhibition, stimulating milk production. Oxytocin triggers the let-down reflex, coordinating milk ejection with infant suckling. Early skin-to-skin contact and frequent feeding strengthen supply through feedback mechanisms. Nurses educate mothers on proper latch, positioning, and feeding intervals, emphasizing that discomfort in early days often reflects adjustment rather than pathology. Engorgement, cracked nipples, or mastitis require prompt assessment and tailored intervention to preserve comfort and continuation of breastfeeding. Breast care involves gentle cleansing, supportive garments, and avoidance of excessive stimulation when not feeding. Beyond physiology, lactation symbolizes bonding and empowerment—a visible bridge between maternal generosity and newborn survival. In diverse cultural settings, nurses must balance tradition with evidence, validating personal preferences while promoting safe and successful feeding practices. Effective breast care nurtures not only nutrition but also trust and emotional well-being.

Maternal Mental Health and Emotional Adjustment

The psychological transition following childbirth is profound, encompassing hormonal fluctuation, sleep deprivation, and shifting identity. Many women experience transient "baby blues," characterized by tearfulness and mood lability that resolve within two weeks. However, persistent sadness, detachment, or intrusive thoughts may signal postpartum depression or anxiety requiring professional intervention. Nurses occupy a pivotal position in early recognition through empathetic conversation and observation of affect, sleep, and engagement with the infant. Supportive listening, reassurance, and referral when necessary preserve mental health and family stability. Evidence-based guidelines advocate routine screening using validated tools within the postpartum period. Stigma often deters disclosure, making compassionate inquiry crucial. Addressing emotional health alongside physical recovery reaffirms that wellness is indivisible. The nurse's attentiveness not only prevents crisis but restores balance, allowing the mother to integrate her new identity with confidence. Maternal mental health is therefore not an adjunct to care—it is the emotional heartbeat sustaining family resilience.

Postpartum Nutrition and Physical Restoration

Nutrition during the postpartum period fuels healing, lactation, and energy restoration. Increased caloric needs—particularly for breastfeeding women—require balanced intake of protein, iron, calcium, and fluids. Cultural dietary practices influence meal choices, and nurses should assess beliefs to ensure nutritional adequacy without imposing disruption. Hydration supports milk synthesis and metabolic recovery, while micronutrients such as folate and vitamin D sustain maternal immunity. Gradual reintroduction of activity, guided by comfort and medical advice, promotes circulation and emotional well-being. Postpartum exercise improves mood and muscle tone but must respect the body's healing pace. Counseling includes guidance on weight stabilization and realistic expectations about body image. Nutrition is both biological and cultural; thus, individualized planning ensures adherence. Nurses encourage family participation in meal preparation and rest scheduling to alleviate maternal fatigue. Postpartum nutrition, viewed holistically, nourishes not just tissue repair but confidence, vitality, and readiness for the responsibilities of nurturing new life.

Immediate Newborn Transition and Adaptation

At birth, the newborn undergoes rapid physiologic changes essential for independent survival. Pulmonary expansion replaces placental gas exchange, requiring prompt clearance of fluid and establishment of regular breathing. Circulatory adjustments follow—closure of the ductus arteriosus, foramen ovale, and ductus venosus redirect blood flow for oxygenation. Nurses assess Apgar scores, respiratory effort, and tone within minutes, initiating warmth, stimulation, and airway maintenance as indicated. Skin-to-skin contact stabilizes temperature and glucose levels while fostering bonding. Delayed cord clamping enhances neonatal iron stores without increasing risk. Observing color, cry, and reflexes provides continuous feedback about adaptation. Every newborn, regardless of risk, demands vigilant surveillance during the first hours of life. Compassion complements competence—gentle handling and reassuring communication soothe parental anxiety. The transition to extrauterine life exemplifies the seamless collaboration between physiology and care, as each observation, touch, and word contributes to the infant's safe arrival into the continuum of human connection.

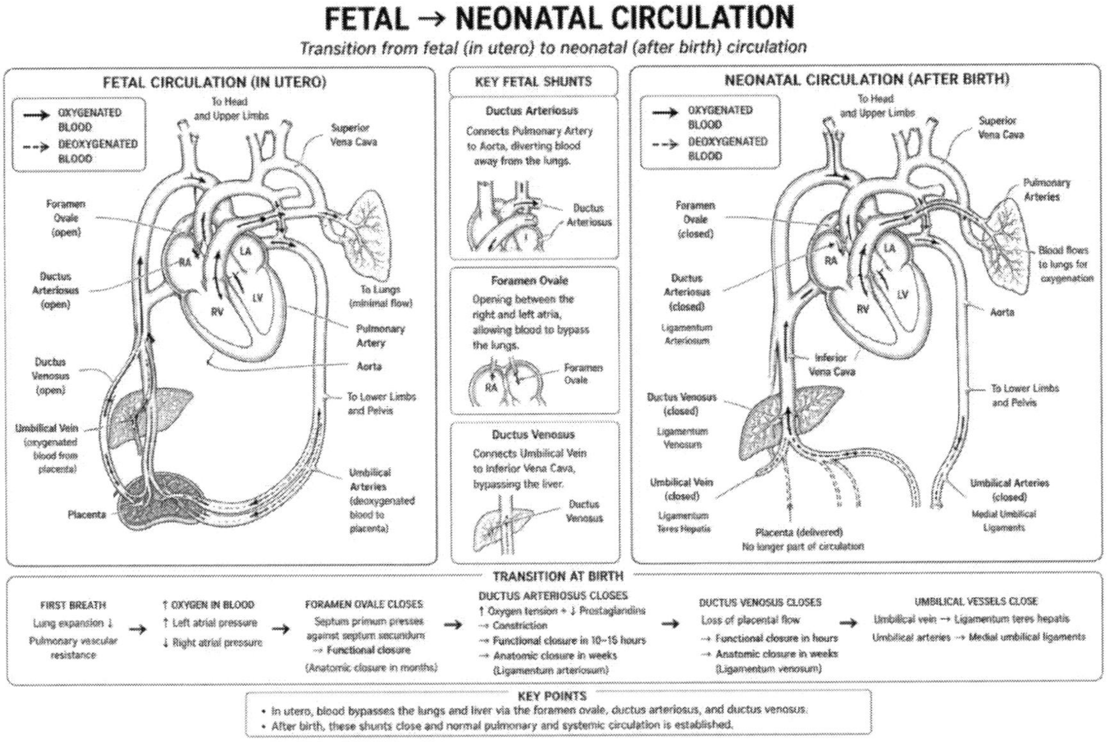

Thermoregulation and Early Skin-to-Skin Care

Thermal stability is one of the newborn's most critical physiological challenges. At birth, the transition from the warm intrauterine environment to cooler external air can rapidly result in heat loss through evaporation, convection, conduction, and radiation. Hypothermia increases oxygen consumption, glucose depletion, and metabolic acidosis, all of which compromise adaptation. Immediate drying and placement of the newborn on the mother's chest prevent these losses through conduction and the natural warmth of maternal skin. Skin-to-skin contact also promotes colonization with maternal flora, stabilizes respiration, and supports breastfeeding initiation. The nurse's vigilance in temperature monitoring, appropriate clothing, and environmental control maintains thermal safety. When radiant warmers or incubators are necessary, gentle handling and minimal exposure protect fragile thermoregulation mechanisms. Skin-to-skin care, often termed "kangaroo care," embodies both science and affection—it transforms physiological necessity into nurturing intimacy, reinforcing the inseparable bond between warmth and survival.

Neonatal Respiratory and Cardiovascular Assessment

Effective transition to independent breathing defines neonatal vitality. The newborn's first cry marks the aeration of the lungs and establishment of functional residual capacity. Nurses assess respiratory rate, rhythm, and the presence of grunting or retractions, which may indicate distress. Cardiovascular adaptation follows rapidly, with closure of fetal shunts and stabilization of systemic circulation. Heart rate should remain between 100 and 160 beats per minute, though transient fluctuations occur as the infant adapts. Delayed cord clamping, supported by current evidence, enhances blood volume and iron stores, improving oxygen delivery in early life. Continuous observation during the first hour ensures prompt detection of cyanosis, irregular pulse, or murmurs. Gentle tactile stimulation and maintenance of airway patency remain first-line interventions for mild compromise. Nurses integrate physiological understanding with compassionate presence, ensuring that every breath and heartbeat receives not only medical scrutiny but human reassurance—an affirmation that adaptation is proceeding safely and strongly.

Neonatal Nutrition and Feeding Support

Feeding in the neonatal period establishes both physiological stability and emotional security. Colostrum, rich in immunoglobulins and growth factors, provides the first immunologic shield and prepares the gut for nutrient absorption. Exclusive breastfeeding is recommended whenever possible during the first six months, but achieving success requires practical instruction and continuous encouragement. Nurses guide mothers in positioning, recognizing feeding cues, and maintaining regular intervals. When breastfeeding is contraindicated or supplementation necessary, safe formula preparation and sterile handling are taught with equal respect. Observation of latch, swallowing, and weight gain allows early identification of feeding difficulties or dehydration. Beyond mechanics, feeding nurtures relationship—the reciprocal gaze and touch forming the foundation of trust. By supporting mothers through fatigue, uncertainty, and societal pressures, nurses sustain not only the infant's nutrition but also the emotional nourishment that defines human caregiving at its purest form.

Newborn Screening, Immunization, and Early Detection

Early preventive interventions anchor long-term health. Within the first days of life, newborn screening tests identify metabolic, endocrine, and hematologic disorders before symptoms manifest, allowing timely treatment. Procedures such as phenylketonuria screening, bilirubin measurement, and congenital heart disease screening form the foundation of neonatal safety nets. Immunizations—most notably hepatitis B—initiate lifelong protection. The nurse's role includes obtaining informed consent, explaining procedures, and ensuring proper timing and documentation. Pain minimization through swaddling or breastfeeding during heel pricks demonstrates compassionate technique. Early detection also extends to visual, auditory, and developmental assessments, establishing baselines for growth monitoring. Public health frameworks emphasize that these preventive actions embody equity: every infant, regardless of circumstance, deserves the same opportunity for a healthy start. Thus, newborn screening transforms from laboratory process into ethical practice—proactive care that secures the silent promise of wellness before disease can speak.

Infection Prevention and Environmental Hygiene

Newborns possess immature immune systems, making infection control paramount. Simple practices such as hand hygiene, clean cord care, and avoidance of unnecessary invasive procedures prevent life-threatening sepsis. Environmental cleanliness within the maternity ward—sterile instruments, disinfected surfaces, and controlled visitor access—minimizes microbial exposure. The umbilical cord, a potential portal for pathogens, requires dry care unless antiseptic use is indicated by local epidemiology. Nurses educate families on recognizing early signs of infection: fever, lethargy, feeding refusal, or umbilical redness. In resource-limited settings, infection prevention often depends on education as much as equipment. Evidence-based guidelines confirm that infection rates decline when mothers and caregivers participate actively in hygiene maintenance. The nurse's vigilance transforms routine observation into life protection. Infection prevention, though seemingly procedural, reflects deep moral commitment—guarding the fragile line between vulnerability and survival during the newborn's earliest days.

Parental Bonding and Psychosocial Integration

The postpartum period extends beyond physical recovery to encompass the formation of emotional connections that shape family identity. Parental bonding emerges through shared moments of eye contact, voice recognition, and touch. Nurses nurture this process by promoting rooming-in, minimizing separation, and encouraging parental participation in newborn care. Fathers, partners, and extended family members are integral to this adjustment, finding their place within the caregiving circle. Emotional sensitivity is essential, especially for parents coping with exhaustion, uncertainty, or previous trauma. Education in infant cues, soothing techniques, and safe sleep practices empowers confidence. Bonding is not a single event but a continuum of mutual recognition that unfolds with patience and tenderness. When health professionals support emotional connection alongside clinical care, they foster resilient families capable of meeting the demands of early parenting with love and stability—a foundation upon which lifelong attachment and well-being are built.

Discharge Planning and Community Continuity of Care

Safe transition from hospital to home completes the continuum of postpartum and newborn care. Discharge planning begins at admission, integrating clinical readiness, parental competence, and access to community resources. Nurses ensure that mothers understand signs of danger—such as excessive bleeding, fever, or neonatal jaundice—and know when and where to seek help. Education covers breastfeeding, hygiene, immunization schedules, and contraception options. Coordination with public health agencies or home-visiting programs extends support beyond discharge, particularly for high-risk families. Documentation and communication with primary care providers ensure continuity. Cultural sensitivity remains vital: instructions must respect language, literacy, and traditional practices while maintaining evidence-based safety. The goal is empowerment, not dependence—equipping families to navigate the early weeks with confidence. When discharge planning is thorough and compassionate, hospital walls no longer define care boundaries; instead, a seamless network of knowledge and trust accompanies mother and child into the world.

Chapter 5: Professional Practice Issues

Ethical Foundations in Obstetric Nursing

Table: Ethical Principles

Principle	Definition	Example
Autonomy	Patient choice	Informed consent
Beneficence	Do good	Best care
Nonmaleficence	Do no harm	Avoid unnecessary procedures
Justice	Fairness	Equal care

Ethical practice in obstetric nursing unites technical competence with moral responsibility. Every decision, from fetal monitoring to patient education, involves respect for autonomy, beneficence, nonmaleficence, and justice. Nurses often navigate dual accountability to both mother and fetus, a balance that demands nuanced reasoning. Confidentiality, truth-telling, and informed consent are daily moral tests, especially when cultural or religious beliefs intersect with medical advice. Ethical frameworks guide practitioners through dilemmas such as refusal of treatment, end-of-life decisions in perinatal loss, or differing interpretations of fetal viability. Reflection, peer dialogue, and adherence to institutional ethics committees sustain integrity under pressure. Compassion and fairness define professionalism more than certainty does; nurses who listen before acting embody true ethical competence. In every obstetric unit, ethics are not abstract philosophy—they are lived moments where empathy meets accountability, shaping the safety, dignity, and trust that form the soul of nursing practice.

Legal Responsibility and Accountability

The legal framework of obstetric nursing protects both patient rights and professional integrity. Documentation accuracy, adherence to institutional policies, and evidence-based interventions form the foundation of defensible practice. Legal accountability extends beyond technical error to include omission, negligence, or failure to communicate significant findings. Informed consent is a cornerstone: nurses ensure that patients understand procedures, alternatives, and potential risks before participation. Mandatory reporting laws govern specific circumstances such as abuse, infectious disease, or impaired practitioners, reflecting nursing's duty to safeguard the vulnerable. When adverse outcomes occur, the nurse's contemporaneous notes become vital legal evidence. Ethical and legal standards intersect through the principle of fidelity—honoring the promises inherent in professional commitment. Obstetric nursing, often involving high-stakes decisions under time constraints, requires vigilance, documentation precision, and continual competence renewal. In law as in ethics, transparency and honesty remain the strongest shields for both patient and practitioner.

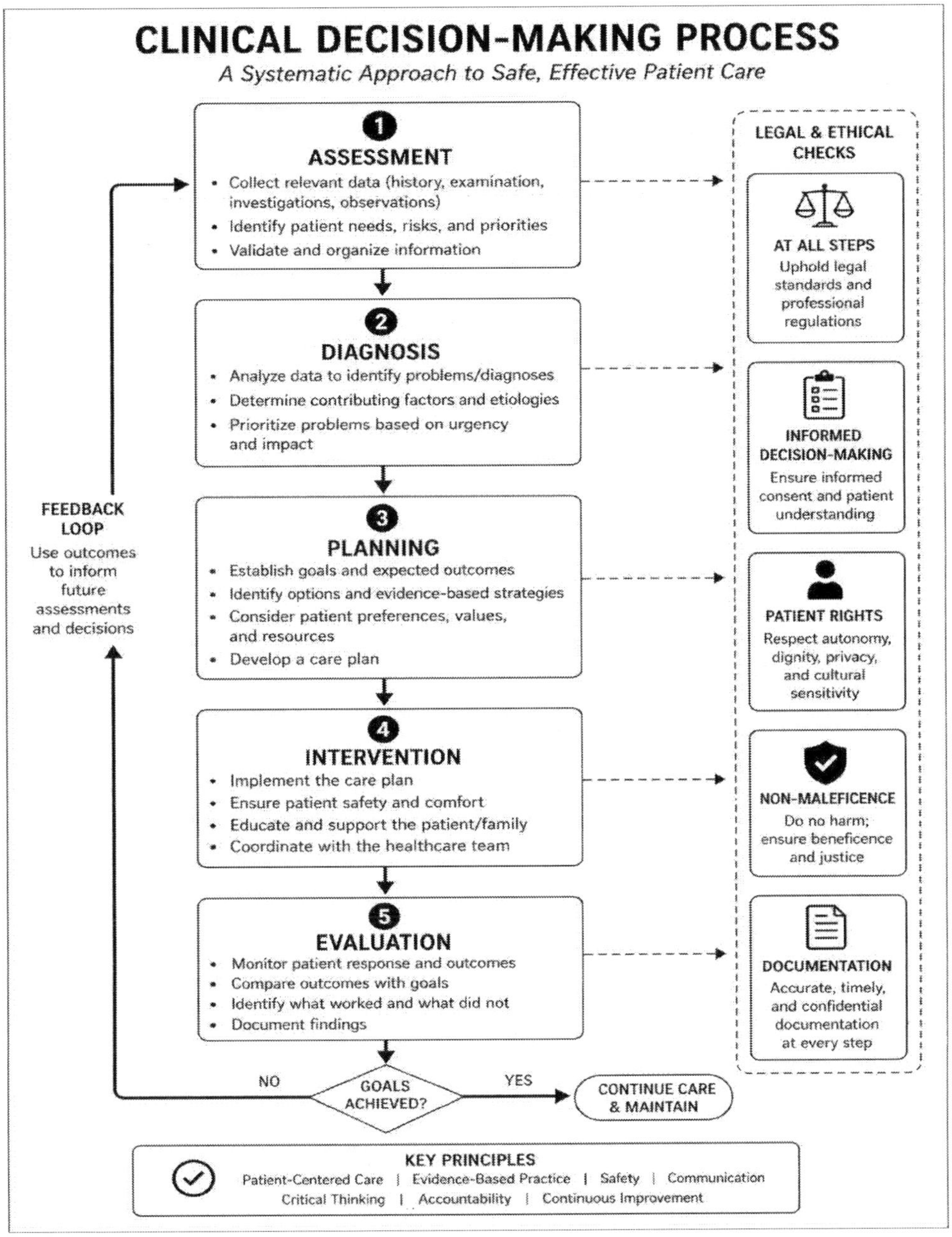

Interprofessional Collaboration and Team Communication

Safe obstetric care depends on coordinated teamwork among nurses, midwives, physicians, anesthetists, and neonatal specialists. Clear communication transforms individual expertise into collective safety. Structured frameworks such as SBAR (Situation, Background, Assessment, Recommendation) minimize misunderstandings during handoffs and emergencies. The nurse often serves as the communication hub, synthesizing patient data and conveying updates across disciplines. Interprofessional collaboration thrives in environments of mutual respect, where hierarchy yields to shared purpose. Research consistently links teamwork quality with reduced error rates and improved maternal outcomes. Beyond spoken exchange, collaboration includes emotional intelligence—reading nonverbal cues, acknowledging stress, and fostering calm during crises. Debriefing after complex deliveries sustains psychological resilience and learning. The obstetric nurse embodies both advocate and mediator, ensuring that every professional voice contributes to the unified goal of safe, compassionate birth. Collaboration, at its core, is not about authority but about harmony in pursuit of life.

Leadership, Delegation, and Professional Growth

Leadership in nursing extends far beyond managerial authority—it reflects the ability to inspire confidence, prioritize effectively, and model accountability. In the labor and delivery setting, leaders coordinate patient flow, anticipate complications, and mentor novice staff under intense conditions. Delegation requires understanding scope of practice and ensuring that each team member functions within competency limits. Clear direction paired with trust transforms delegation into empowerment rather than control. Continuous professional development—through certification, education, and reflective practice—sustains competence in evolving obstetric standards. Leadership also includes moral courage: the willingness to question unsafe orders, advocate for resources, and defend patient dignity. Effective leaders cultivate cultures where inquiry and improvement replace blame. In obstetric nursing, where every decision may influence two lives, leadership is not optional—it is a moral imperative expressed through presence, precision, and unwavering professionalism in every clinical encounter.

Cultural Competence and Patient Advocacy

Cultural competence stands at the heart of patient-centered obstetric care. Pregnancy and birth are profoundly influenced by cultural values, language, and belief systems that shape expectations and decision-making. Nurses act as cultural translators, bridging differences with sensitivity and respect. Advocacy begins with listening—understanding how each patient defines safety, comfort, and family participation. When cultural practices conflict with medical recommendations, dialogue grounded in empathy preserves trust while protecting health. Professional advocacy also encompasses equity, ensuring access to pain relief, consent comprehension, and unbiased care for all demographics. In diverse communities, nurses become both caregivers and cultural navigators, defending patients' rights to informed choice without judgment. True advocacy blends scientific reasoning with cultural humility, affirming that dignity is not granted by policy but by respect. Through cultural awareness, obstetric nurses honor the universality of birth while celebrating the individuality of every family's story.

Professional Integrity and Reflective Practice

Integrity defines the moral backbone of nursing. It encompasses honesty in documentation, authenticity in communication, and accountability for one's actions. Reflective practice—the deliberate review of experiences—enables nurses to transform challenges into insight. In obstetrics, where decisions carry profound emotional weight, self-reflection nurtures emotional resilience and ethical clarity. Discussing complex cases, analyzing errors without fear, and seeking mentorship sustain professional growth. Maintaining boundaries, safeguarding confidentiality, and upholding evidence-based standards reflect inner discipline. Integrity is also collective: it flourishes in teams that value truth and learning over blame. Continuous reflection prevents complacency, ensuring that technical skill remains aligned with compassion. As obstetric nurses witness both life's beginnings and its fragility, integrity becomes their constant compass. It reminds the profession that excellence is not only what is done, but how it is done—with honesty, empathy, and unwavering respect for the trust placed in their care.

Chapter 6 – Practice Questions

Question (1-100)

Q1. A pregnant woman at 30 weeks presents with elevated blood pressure and proteinuria on examination. What is the most likely diagnosis?
(A) Chronic hypertension
(B) Eclampsia
(C) Preeclampsia
(D) Gestational hypertension
Q2. A woman with preeclampsia develops convulsions at 34 weeks of gestation. What condition does this indicate?
(A) Severe hypertension
(B) Cerebral hemorrhage
(C) HELLP syndrome
(D) Eclampsia
Q3. A pregnant patient with poorly controlled diabetes has an increased risk of which fetal outcome?
(A) Premature closure of ductus
(B) Growth restriction
(C) Skeletal anomalies
(D) Macrosomia
Q4. A pregnant woman presents with painless vaginal bleeding during the third trimester without uterine tenderness. What is the likely diagnosis?
(A) Placenta previa
(B) Uterine rupture
(C) Cervical dilation
(D) Placental abruption
Q5. A pregnant woman at 36 weeks presents with vaginal bleeding, abdominal pain, and a tender uterus. What is the most likely diagnosis?
(A) Preterm labor
(B) Cervical insufficiency
(C) Placental abruption
(D) Placenta previa
Q6. A woman carrying twins is being monitored closely during pregnancy. What complication is she at higher risk for?
(A) Post-term pregnancy
(B) Preterm labor
(C) Reduced uterine activity
(D) Decreased fetal growth
Q7. A pregnant woman undergoes a test to evaluate fetal heart rate response to movements without uterine contractions. What test is being performed?
(A) Nonstress test
(B) Doppler study
(C) Biophysical profile
(D) Contraction stress test
Q8. A fetus is assessed using ultrasound and scoring includes breathing, movement, tone, and amniotic fluid. What test is this?
(A) Biophysical profile

(B) NST only
(C) Doppler velocimetry
(D) Contraction test

Q9. During fetal monitoring, a baseline heart rate of 120 bpm is recorded. How is this interpreted?
(A) Tachycardia
(B) Abnormal variability
(C) Bradycardia
(D) Normal baseline

Q10. A pregnant woman presents with fever, uterine tenderness, and foul-smelling discharge. What is the most likely diagnosis?
(A) Ectopic pregnancy
(B) Urinary infection
(C) Placenta previa
(D) Chorioamnionitis

Q11. A pregnant woman presents at 28 weeks with persistent headache, visual disturbances, and elevated blood pressure readings. What is the priority assessment finding?
(A) Degree of proteinuria
(B) Signs of neurological involvement
(C) Presence of edema
(D) Fundal height measurement

Q12. A pregnant patient is found to have hemoglobin significantly below normal levels during routine screening. What is the most likely hematologic condition?
(A) Thrombocytopenia
(B) Polycythemia
(C) Anemia
(D) Leukocytosis

Q13. A patient at 34 weeks reports decreased fetal movements. Initial nonstress test is non-reactive. What is the next appropriate step?
(A) Immediate delivery
(B) Repeat NST later
(C) Perform biophysical profile
(D) Start induction

Q14. A pregnant woman presents with vaginal bleeding and signs of shock including low blood pressure and tachycardia. What is the immediate priority?
(A) Conduct pelvic exam
(B) Administer antibiotics
(C) Initiate IV fluids
(D) Perform ultrasound

Q15. A pregnant patient with infection presents with fever, abdominal pain, and uterine tenderness. What complication should be suspected?
(A) Hyperemesis gravidarum
(B) Ectopic pregnancy
(C) Chorioamnionitis
(D) Placenta previa

Q16. A woman with history of substance use presents during pregnancy. What is the most important initial approach?
(A) Immediate reporting
(B) Discharge from care

(C) Nonjudgmental assessment
(D) Strict isolation

Q17. A pregnant patient presents with contractions and cervical changes at 33 weeks gestation. What condition is most likely?
(A) Post-term labor
(B) Term labor
(C) Preterm labor
(D) False labor

Q18. A fetus shows absent variability on electronic fetal monitoring. What does this indicate?
(A) Maternal dehydration
(B) Possible fetal distress
(C) Normal finding
(D) Fetal well-being

Q19. A pregnant woman is diagnosed with placenta previa. What activity should be avoided to prevent complications?
(A) Blood pressure monitoring
(B) Walking
(C) Ultrasound scanning
(D) Digital vaginal examination

Q20. A pregnant patient presents with severe abdominal pain and rigid uterus without external bleeding. What is the likely diagnosis?
(A) Placenta previa
(B) Cervical dilation
(C) Urinary infection
(D) Placental abruption

Q21. A pregnant woman develops high blood pressure after 20 weeks without proteinuria or organ dysfunction. What is the diagnosis?
(A) Chronic hypertension
(B) Preeclampsia
(C) Eclampsia
(D) Gestational hypertension

Q22. A pregnant patient complains of blurred vision and severe headache with elevated blood pressure. Which complication is most concerning?
(A) Liver dysfunction
(B) Renal impairment
(C) Neurological involvement
(D) Cardiac changes

Q23. A woman at 31 weeks gestation presents with regular contractions and cervical dilation. What is the most appropriate initial classification?
(A) Latent phase labor
(B) False labor
(C) Preterm labor
(D) Term labor

Q24. A pregnant patient with suspected infection has fever, foul discharge, and uterine tenderness. What is the primary concern?
(A) Urinary tract infection
(B) Respiratory infection
(C) Intrauterine infection

(D) Gastrointestinal illness

Q25. A fetus shows no accelerations on nonstress testing despite movement stimulation. What does this indicate?

(A) Normal finding
(B) Reactive pattern
(C) Non-reactive pattern
(D) Hyperactive fetus

Q26. A pregnant woman presents with vaginal bleeding, abdominal pain, and signs of shock. What is the immediate management priority?

(A) Obtain detailed history
(B) Perform ultrasound
(C) Stabilize circulation
(D) Start oral medications

Q27. A woman in pregnancy reports reduced fetal movements over the past day. What is the most appropriate first assessment?

(A) Nonstress test
(B) Surgical intervention
(C) Medication therapy
(D) Immediate delivery

Q28. A pregnant patient has severe anemia affecting oxygen transport. What is the primary maternal risk?

(A) Excess fluid retention
(B) Increased blood viscosity
(C) Elevated blood pressure
(D) Reduced oxygen delivery

Q29. A fetus demonstrates moderate variability on monitoring. What does this finding indicate?

(A) Fetal distress
(B) Hypoxia
(C) Normal status
(D) Acidosis

Q30. A pregnant woman with multiple gestation is monitored for complications. What is the most likely issue due to uterine overdistension?

(A) Preterm contractions
(B) Reduced blood volume
(C) Post-term pregnancy
(D) Decreased fetal activity

Q31. A pregnant woman presents with vaginal bleeding in early pregnancy along with abdominal pain and fainting episodes. What condition should be strongly suspected?

(A) Threatened abortion
(B) Complete abortion
(C) Molar pregnancy
(D) Ectopic pregnancy

Q32. A pregnant patient with heavy vaginal bleeding has a dilated cervix and partial expulsion of products of conception. What is the most likely diagnosis?

(A) Missed abortion
(B) Complete abortion
(C) Threatened abortion
(D) Incomplete abortion

Q33. A pregnant woman presents with signs of shock including low blood pressure, rapid pulse, and cold clammy skin. What is the primary clinical concern?
(A) Hemorrhage
(B) Dehydration
(C) Infection
(D) Hypertension
Q34. A pregnant patient with fever and purulent vaginal discharge is evaluated. What underlying issue is most likely present?
(A) Urinary infection
(B) Pelvic infection
(C) Skin infection
(D) Respiratory infection
Q35. A woman presents with light vaginal bleeding, a closed cervix, and a uterus consistent with gestational age. What is the most likely diagnosis?
(A) Threatened abortion
(B) Incomplete abortion
(C) Molar pregnancy
(D) Ectopic pregnancy
Q36. A pregnant woman has heavy bleeding and a uterus larger than expected with no detectable fetus. What condition should be considered?
(A) Complete abortion
(B) Ectopic pregnancy
(C) Molar pregnancy
(D) Threatened abortion
Q37. A pregnant patient presents with abdominal pain and rebound tenderness along with fever. What complication should be suspected?
(A) Placenta previa
(B) Infection
(C) Hypertension
(D) Preterm labor
Q38. A pregnant woman has a history of expulsion of products of conception with minimal bleeding afterward. What is the most likely diagnosis?
(A) Molar pregnancy
(B) Complete abortion
(C) Incomplete abortion
(D) Threatened abortion
Q39. A pregnant patient is being evaluated for early pregnancy bleeding. What diagnostic tool is essential for confirming the cause?
(A) Urine analysis
(B) Temperature recording
(C) Blood pressure measurement
(D) Ultrasound examination
Q40. A pregnant woman presents with signs of infection and foul-smelling discharge after pregnancy loss. What complication is most likely?
(A) Sepsis
(B) Preterm labor
(C) Hypertension
(D) Placenta previa

Q41. A pregnant woman presents with abdominal pain, distension, and shoulder pain along with signs of internal bleeding. What is the most likely diagnosis?
(A) Urinary infection
(B) Ectopic pregnancy
(C) Threatened abortion
(D) Complete abortion
Q42. A pregnant patient presents with heavy vaginal bleeding where a pad is soaked within minutes and large clots are passed. How is this bleeding classified?
(A) Light bleeding
(B) Heavy bleeding
(C) Moderate bleeding
(D) Intermittent bleeding
Q43. A woman presents with vaginal bleeding and a uterus smaller than expected for gestational age. What condition is most consistent with this finding?
(A) Complete abortion
(B) Incomplete abortion
(C) Molar pregnancy
(D) Ectopic pregnancy
Q44. A pregnant patient is evaluated for possible ectopic pregnancy. Why should bimanual examination be performed gently?
(A) To prevent rupture
(B) To assess cervix
(C) To improve diagnosis
(D) To reduce discomfort
Q45. A pregnant woman presents with signs of infection including fever, malaise, and foul vaginal discharge after abortion. What is the likely complication?
(A) Sepsis
(B) Hypertension
(C) Preterm labor
(D) Placenta previa
Q46. A pregnant patient shows signs of shock but no obvious external bleeding is observed. What should be considered?
(A) Internal bleeding
(B) Infection only
(C) Dehydration
(D) Normal variation
Q47. A woman presents with light bleeding and mild cramping in early pregnancy, with cervix remaining closed. What is the expected management approach?
(A) Induction of labor
(B) Observation and monitoring
(C) Immediate surgery
(D) Antibiotic therapy
Q48. A pregnant patient presents with abdominal pain, fever, and signs of peritonitis. What is the most serious underlying concern?
(A) Gastrointestinal upset
(B) Mild infection
(C) Severe intra-abdominal infection
(D) Normal pregnancy discomfort

Q49. A pregnant woman presents with vaginal bleeding and cervix dilated but no expulsion of products yet. What condition does this represent?
(A) Complete abortion
(B) Missed abortion
(C) Threatened abortion
(D) Inevitable abortion
Q50. A pregnant patient is suspected to have fetal distress based on abnormal fetal heart rate findings. What range indicates abnormality?
(A) 110-160 bpm
(B) 100-120 bpm
(C) 120-140 bpm
(D) Less than 100 or greater than 180 bpm
Q51. A pregnant woman presents with rapid pulse, low blood pressure, and confusion. What clinical state is indicated?
(A) Hypertension
(B) Dehydration
(C) Shock
(D) Infection
Q52. A pregnant patient reports painful urination, fever, and weakness during evaluation. What condition should be considered?
(A) Respiratory infection
(B) Skin infection
(C) Urinary tract infection
(D) Neurological disorder
Q53. A pregnant woman presents with severe abdominal tenderness, fever, and shallow breathing. What is the likely concern?
(A) Serious infection
(B) Musculoskeletal pain
(C) Mild discomfort
(D) Normal pregnancy change
Q54. A pregnant patient presents with respiratory distress and bluish discoloration of the skin. What is the most critical assessment focus?
(A) Fluid intake
(B) Nutritional status
(C) Oxygenation status
(D) Activity level
Q55. A pregnant woman presents with frequent painful contractions and blood-stained mucus discharge. What does this suggest?
(A) Infection
(B) Hypertension
(C) Urinary problem
(D) Labor onset
Q56. A pregnant patient reports rupture of membranes and onset of contractions. What is the immediate clinical implication?
(A) Assess labor progress
(B) Start antibiotics
(C) Delay evaluation
(D) Discharge patient

Q57. A pregnant woman presents with severe headache, blurred vision, and vomiting. What condition should be considered urgently?
(A) Neurological complication
(B) Muscular strain
(C) Gastrointestinal illness
(D) Skin disorder
Q58. A pregnant patient appears pale and reports weakness and fainting episodes. What underlying issue is most likely?
(A) Hypertension
(B) Hyperactivity
(C) Anemia
(D) Infection
Q59. A pregnant woman presents with vaginal bleeding and uterus atony after childbirth. What is the likely cause?
(A) Infection
(B) Hypertension
(C) Hemorrhage
(D) Dehydration
Q60. A pregnant patient presents with fever, neck stiffness, and altered consciousness. What is the most serious concern?
(A) Severe systemic infection
(B) Muscular issue
(C) Mild infection
(D) Normal variation
Q61. A pregnant woman at 10 weeks presents with lower abdominal pain, dizziness, and light vaginal bleeding. On examination, she appears pale and hypotensive. What is the most likely diagnosis?
(A) Urinary infection
(B) Threatened abortion
(C) Complete abortion
(D) Ectopic pregnancy
Q62. A pregnant patient presents with heavy vaginal bleeding, dilated cervix, and no expulsion of tissue yet. She reports increasing cramping pain. What condition is most consistent with this presentation?
(A) Threatened abortion
(B) Inevitable abortion
(C) Complete abortion
(D) Molar pregnancy
Q63. A pregnant woman arrives with fever, foul-smelling discharge, and severe lower abdominal tenderness following a recent abortion. What is the most appropriate immediate concern?
(A) Hypertension
(B) Normal recovery
(C) Mild infection
(D) Sepsis
Q64. A pregnant patient at 20 weeks presents with vaginal bleeding and reports that her uterus feels smaller than expected. She also reports previous passage of tissue. What is the likely diagnosis?
(A) Threatened abortion
(B) Complete abortion
(C) Ectopic pregnancy

(D) Incomplete abortion

Q65. A pregnant woman presents with abdominal pain, rebound tenderness, fever, and rigid abdomen. Her condition is worsening rapidly. What is the most serious underlying issue?

(A) Muscular pain
(B) Peritonitis
(C) Mild infection
(D) Urinary infection

Q66. A pregnant woman presents with vaginal bleeding, a closed cervix, and mild cramping. Ultrasound shows a viable pregnancy. What is the best classification of her condition?

(A) Threatened abortion
(B) Incomplete abortion
(C) Molar pregnancy
(D) Inevitable abortion

Q67. A pregnant patient develops sudden abdominal pain and signs of shock without visible bleeding. What hidden complication should be considered?

(A) Dehydration
(B) Mild cramping
(C) Infection
(D) Internal hemorrhage

Q68. A pregnant woman presents with high fever, weakness, and purulent vaginal discharge. What is the most appropriate initial management step?

(A) Delay treatment
(B) Observation only
(C) Start antibiotics
(D) Discharge home

Q69. A pregnant patient is evaluated for early bleeding and ultrasound shows no fetal activity with abnormal tissue growth. The uterus is larger than expected. What is the most likely diagnosis?

(A) Threatened abortion
(B) Complete abortion
(C) Ectopic pregnancy
(D) Molar pregnancy

Q70. A pregnant woman presents with heavy bleeding, dilated cervix, and partial expulsion of tissue. She continues to bleed significantly. What is the likely diagnosis?

(A) Ectopic pregnancy
(B) Complete abortion
(C) Threatened abortion
(D) Incomplete abortion

Q71. A pregnant woman presents with cyanosis and difficulty breathing during assessment. What is the most immediate concern?

(A) Cardiac output issue
(B) Fluid imbalance
(C) Impaired oxygenation
(D) Nutritional deficiency

Q72. A pregnant patient is found to have temperature above 38°C with lethargy and painful urination. What is the likely diagnosis?

(A) Respiratory infection
(B) Neurological disorder
(C) Urinary tract infection

(D) Skin infection

Q73. A pregnant woman presents with abdominal pain and low blood pressure along with a rapid pulse. What should be suspected first?

(A) Mild discomfort
(B) Dehydration
(C) Shock
(D) Hypertension

Q74. A pregnant patient reports sudden onset abdominal pain and rigid abdomen with signs of distress. No external bleeding is noted. What is the most likely cause?

(A) Normal discomfort
(B) Placenta previa
(C) Urinary infection
(D) Concealed hemorrhage

Q75. A pregnant woman presents with foul-smelling vaginal discharge, fever, and general weakness. What is the most appropriate initial action?

(A) Provide reassurance
(B) Start antibiotics
(C) Observe condition
(D) Delay treatment

Q76. A pregnant patient presents with mild vaginal bleeding and a closed cervix without significant pain. What condition is most consistent?

(A) Complete abortion
(B) Incomplete abortion
(C) Threatened abortion
(D) Inevitable abortion

Q77. A pregnant woman arrives with severe abdominal pain, fever, and rebound tenderness. Her condition deteriorates quickly. What serious complication should be suspected?

(A) Muscle strain
(B) Peritonitis
(C) Normal change
(D) Mild infection

Q78. A pregnant patient presents with heavy bleeding, dilated cervix, and ongoing expulsion of tissue. What is the most appropriate diagnosis?

(A) Complete abortion
(B) Ectopic pregnancy
(C) Incomplete abortion
(D) Threatened abortion

Q79. A pregnant woman presents with vaginal bleeding and reports that her uterus feels larger than expected. No fetal heart is detected. What condition should be suspected?

(A) Urinary infection
(B) Molar pregnancy
(C) Complete abortion
(D) Threatened abortion

Q80. A pregnant patient presents with vaginal bleeding, abdominal pain, and signs of shock. Immediate stabilization is initiated. What is the next important step after stabilization?

(A) Discharge patient
(B) Delay further care
(C) Provide reassurance

(D) Identify underlying cause

Q81. A pregnant woman presents with difficulty breathing, wheezing, and pallor on examination. What is the primary system affected?

(A) Musculoskeletal system
(B) Gastrointestinal system
(C) Cardiovascular system
(D) Respiratory system

Q82. A pregnant patient presents with cool clammy skin, weak pulse, and systolic blood pressure below 90 mmHg. What condition is indicated?

(A) Infection only
(B) Shock
(C) Mild dehydration
(D) Hypertension

Q83. A pregnant woman presents with vaginal bleeding, and the placenta has not been delivered after childbirth. What is the likely concern?

(A) Respiratory distress
(B) Urinary infection
(C) Normal recovery
(D) Retained placenta

Q84. A pregnant patient reports fever, neck stiffness, and shallow breathing. What is the most serious implication of these findings?

(A) Severe infection
(B) Normal variation
(C) Muscle fatigue
(D) Mild illness

Q85. A pregnant woman presents with abdominal pain and is found to have low blood pressure and rapid pulse. What is the priority nursing action?

(A) Delay treatment
(B) Begin fluid resuscitation
(C) Provide oral medication
(D) Discharge patient

Q86. A pregnant patient presents with fever, tender abdomen, and purulent discharge from the genital tract. What condition should be suspected?

(A) Pelvic infection
(B) Skin infection
(C) Respiratory infection
(D) Cardiac condition

Q87. A pregnant woman reports fainting episodes and appears weak and pale during examination. What is the most likely underlying issue?

(A) Hypertension
(B) Anemia
(C) Infection
(D) Hyperactivity

Q88. A pregnant patient presents with vaginal bleeding and is asked about gestational age and recent delivery. Why is this information important?

(A) To identify cause of bleeding
(B) To check activity level
(C) To evaluate sleep pattern

(D) To assess nutrition

Q89. A pregnant woman presents with severe abdominal pain and a rigid uterus along with signs of shock. What is the likely diagnosis?

(A) Placenta previa
(B) Urinary infection
(C) Placental abruption
(D) Normal contraction

Q90. A pregnant patient presents with fever, painful urination, and weakness. What is the most appropriate initial step?

(A) Provide reassurance
(B) Ignore symptoms
(C) Delay assessment
(D) Evaluate for infection

Q91. A pregnant woman presents with cyanosis, shallow breathing, and restlessness during assessment. What is the immediate priority action?

(A) Evaluate nutritional intake
(B) Assess oxygenation status
(C) Review medical history
(D) Check urinary output

Q92. A pregnant patient presents with fast weak pulse and cold clammy skin along with hypotension. What condition is most consistent with these findings?

(A) Normal adaptation
(B) Hypertension
(C) Infection
(D) Shock

Q93. A pregnant woman reports fever, frequent urination, and pain during urination. What is the most likely diagnosis?

(A) Urinary tract infection
(B) Skin infection
(C) Respiratory infection
(D) Gastrointestinal illness

Q94. A pregnant patient presents with vaginal bleeding and is asked whether she recently gave birth or is currently pregnant. What is the purpose of this question?

(A) To assess emotional status
(B) To evaluate diet history
(C) To assess activity level
(D) To determine bleeding cause

Q95. A pregnant woman presents with severe abdominal pain, rapid pulse, and low blood pressure. What is the most likely clinical condition?

(A) Hypertension
(B) Mild discomfort
(C) Shock
(D) Infection

Q96. A pregnant patient presents with fever, abdominal tenderness, and purulent vaginal discharge. What is the most likely underlying issue?

(A) Pelvic infection
(B) Skin infection
(C) Cardiac disorder

(D) Respiratory infection

Q97. A pregnant woman appears pale and reports weakness and dizziness during examination. What is the most likely underlying cause?

(A) Anemia
(B) Hypertension
(C) Hyperactivity
(D) Infection

Q98. A pregnant patient presents with vaginal bleeding and uterus atony following delivery. What is the primary concern?

(A) Infection
(B) Hemorrhage
(C) Dehydration
(D) Hypertension

Q99. A pregnant woman presents with neck stiffness, fever, and altered mental status. What is the most serious implication?

(A) Mild illness
(B) Severe systemic infection
(C) Muscular strain
(D) Normal variation

Q100. A pregnant patient presents with vaginal bleeding and abdominal pain during evaluation. What is the most important initial step in management?

(A) Rapid assessment
(B) Provide reassurance
(C) Delay treatment
(D) Discharge patient

Answer Key and Explanation (1-100)

Q1. Answer: C

Explanation: Preeclampsia is characterized by new-onset hypertension after 20 weeks of gestation accompanied by proteinuria. It results from abnormal placental implantation leading to systemic endothelial dysfunction. The presence of proteinuria distinguishes it from gestational hypertension. Early recognition is important to prevent complications such as eclampsia and organ damage. Close monitoring of maternal and fetal status is essential. ##

Q2. Answer: D

Explanation: Eclampsia is diagnosed when seizures occur in a patient with preeclampsia and cannot be attributed to other causes. It represents a progression of hypertensive disease in pregnancy. The seizures are related to cerebral edema and vascular instability. Immediate management is required to prevent maternal and fetal morbidity. Magnesium sulfate is used to control and prevent further seizures. ##

Q3. Answer: D

Explanation: Maternal hyperglycemia leads to increased glucose transfer to the fetus, stimulating insulin production. Fetal hyperinsulinemia promotes excessive growth and fat deposition. This results in macrosomia, which increases risks during delivery. It may lead to shoulder dystocia and birth trauma. Proper glucose control reduces these complications. ##

Q4. Answer: A

Explanation: Placenta previa presents with painless vaginal bleeding in late pregnancy due to placental placement over the cervical os. The absence of uterine tenderness helps differentiate it from placental abruption. Bleeding occurs as the cervix begins to dilate. Ultrasound is used to confirm the diagnosis. Digital vaginal examination should be avoided to prevent severe hemorrhage. ##

Q5. Answer: C

Explanation: Placental abruption involves premature separation of the placenta from the uterine wall. It typically presents with painful vaginal bleeding and uterine tenderness. The condition compromises fetal oxygenation and may lead to maternal hemorrhage. Risk factors include hypertension and trauma. Immediate evaluation and management are required. ##

Q6. Answer: B

Explanation: Multiple gestation increases the risk of preterm labor due to uterine overdistension. The stretched uterus may initiate contractions earlier than expected. This leads to a higher likelihood of premature birth. Preterm delivery is associated with neonatal complications. Close antenatal monitoring is essential in such pregnancies. ##

Q7. Answer: A

Explanation: The nonstress test evaluates fetal heart rate accelerations in response to fetal movement. It reflects fetal oxygenation and autonomic function. A reactive test indicates adequate fetal well-being. It is noninvasive and widely used in antenatal care. Abnormal results require further assessment. ##

Q8. Answer: A

Explanation: The biophysical profile combines ultrasound parameters with fetal heart rate assessment. It evaluates fetal breathing movements, tone, activity, and amniotic fluid volume. Each component reflects fetal neurological and physiological status. The total score helps determine fetal well-being. It guides decisions regarding continuation or delivery of pregnancy. ##

Q9. Answer: D

Explanation: A fetal heart rate between 110 and 160 bpm is considered normal. A baseline of 120 bpm falls within this range. This indicates adequate fetal oxygenation and autonomic balance. Continuous monitoring helps identify deviations from normal patterns. Interpretation should include variability and other features. ##

Q10. Answer: D

Explanation: Fever with uterine tenderness and foul discharge suggests intrauterine infection. Chorioamnionitis occurs due to infection of the amniotic fluid and membranes. It is associated with prolonged rupture of membranes and labor. Prompt antibiotic therapy is required to reduce maternal and fetal complications. Delivery may be necessary depending on severity. ##

Q11. Answer: B

Explanation: Neurological symptoms such as headache and visual disturbances indicate severe features of hypertensive disorders. These findings suggest risk of progression to eclampsia. Immediate assessment is required to prevent seizures and complications. While proteinuria and edema are relevant, neurological signs reflect more critical involvement. Fundal height does not address acute maternal risk. ##

Q12. Answer: C

Explanation: Low hemoglobin levels indicate anemia, which is common in pregnancy due to increased plasma volume. It can reduce oxygen delivery to maternal and fetal tissues. Early identification allows for appropriate supplementation and management. Other options involve different blood components not reflected by hemoglobin alone. Proper treatment improves maternal and fetal outcomes. ##

Q13. Answer: C

Explanation: A non-reactive NST requires further evaluation of fetal well-being using a biophysical profile. This provides additional information about fetal oxygenation and neurological status. Immediate delivery is not indicated without further assessment. Repeating NST alone may delay necessary intervention. A comprehensive evaluation helps guide appropriate management decisions. ##

Q14. Answer: C

Explanation: Signs of shock require immediate stabilization with intravenous fluids to restore circulation. Rapid management is critical to prevent maternal deterioration. Diagnostic procedures should follow stabilization. Pelvic examination may worsen bleeding in some conditions. Early intervention improves survival outcomes in obstetric emergencies. ##

Q15. Answer: C

Explanation: Fever with uterine tenderness and abdominal pain suggests intrauterine infection. Chorioamnionitis involves infection of fetal membranes and amniotic fluid. It can lead to maternal and fetal complications if untreated. Prompt antibiotic therapy is necessary. Other options do not present with this combination of infection-related symptoms. ##

Q16. Answer: C

Explanation: A nonjudgmental and respectful approach encourages disclosure and trust. It allows proper assessment of substance use and associated risks. Judgmental attitudes may prevent patients from seeking care. Supportive management improves outcomes for both mother and fetus. Building rapport is essential for effective intervention. ##

Q17. Answer: C

Explanation: Preterm labor is defined as regular uterine contractions with cervical changes before 37 weeks. It increases the risk of neonatal complications due to prematurity. Early recognition allows for interventions such as corticosteroids. False labor does not involve cervical changes. Proper diagnosis guides timely management. ##

Q18. Answer: B

Explanation: Variability reflects fetal autonomic nervous system activity and oxygenation. Absent variability may indicate fetal hypoxia or neurological compromise. It requires immediate evaluation and possible intervention. Normal fetal status is usually associated with moderate variability. Continuous monitoring helps detect such abnormalities early. ##

Q19. Answer: D

Explanation: Digital vaginal examination can trigger severe bleeding in placenta previa due to placental location near the cervix. It is contraindicated until placental position is confirmed. Ultrasound is the preferred diagnostic tool. Routine activities like monitoring do not increase bleeding risk. Avoidance of unnecessary exams prevents complications. ##

Q20. Answer: D

Explanation: Placental abruption can present with concealed bleeding, severe pain, and a rigid uterus. External bleeding may be absent in some cases. It is a life-threatening condition affecting both mother and fetus. Immediate assessment and management are required. Other conditions do not present with this combination of findings. ##

Q21. Answer: D

Explanation: Gestational hypertension is defined as new-onset hypertension after 20 weeks without proteinuria or systemic involvement. It differs from preeclampsia by the absence of additional complications. Monitoring is required as it may progress to preeclampsia. Chronic hypertension is diagnosed before pregnancy or early gestation. Eclampsia involves seizures, which are not present here. ##

Q22. Answer: C

Explanation: Visual disturbances and severe headache indicate central nervous system involvement. These symptoms suggest severe features of hypertensive disorders. They increase the risk of seizures and intracranial complications. Immediate evaluation is required to prevent progression. Other organ systems may be affected, but neurological signs indicate urgent risk. ##

Q23. Answer: C

Explanation: Preterm labor is diagnosed when contractions with cervical changes occur before 37 weeks. This condition increases the risk of neonatal morbidity. Early identification allows for interventions such as corticosteroids. False labor does not involve cervical dilation. Accurate classification guides appropriate management strategies. ##

Q24. Answer: C

Explanation: Fever with uterine tenderness and foul discharge strongly suggests intrauterine infection. This condition can compromise both maternal and fetal health. Prompt treatment is necessary to prevent complications. Other infections do not typically involve uterine tenderness. Early recognition improves outcomes significantly. ##

Q25. Answer: C

Explanation: A non-reactive nonstress test is characterized by absence of accelerations with fetal movement. It may indicate fetal hypoxia or sleep cycle. Further evaluation with additional testing is required. A reactive pattern includes accelerations. This finding warrants closer monitoring to assess fetal well-being. ##

Q26. Answer: C

Explanation: In the presence of shock, stabilizing circulation is the immediate priority. This includes fluid resuscitation and monitoring vital signs. Diagnostic steps follow once the patient is stable. Delay in stabilization increases mortality risk. Early intervention is critical in obstetric emergencies. ##

Q27. Answer: A

Explanation: A nonstress test is a noninvasive initial assessment for fetal well-being. It evaluates fetal heart rate response to movement. Reduced movement may indicate compromised fetal status. Further testing may be required depending on results. Immediate delivery is not indicated without assessment. ##

Q28. Answer: D

Explanation: Anemia reduces hemoglobin levels, impairing oxygen transport to tissues. This affects both maternal and fetal oxygenation. Severe anemia can lead to fatigue and complications during delivery. Management includes supplementation and monitoring. Other options are not directly related to anemia. ##

Q29. Answer: C

Explanation: Moderate variability reflects a well-functioning autonomic nervous system. It is a reassuring sign of adequate oxygenation. Absence or minimal variability raises concern for hypoxia. This parameter is a key component of fetal monitoring. Normal variability supports continued observation rather than intervention. ##

Q30. Answer: A

Explanation: Uterine overdistension in multiple gestation increases the likelihood of preterm contractions. This can lead to early labor and delivery. The stretched uterus becomes more sensitive to contraction triggers. Close monitoring is necessary to manage this risk. Other options are not directly related to uterine distension. ##

Q31. Answer: D

Explanation: Ectopic pregnancy should be suspected in early pregnancy with bleeding, abdominal pain, and signs like fainting. These symptoms suggest possible rupture and internal bleeding. It is a life-threatening condition requiring urgent diagnosis and management. Threatened abortion usually lacks severe systemic symptoms. Molar pregnancy presents differently with uterine enlargement and other findings. ##

Q32. Answer: D

Explanation: Incomplete abortion is characterized by heavy bleeding, a dilated cervix, and partial expulsion of pregnancy tissue. Retained products continue to cause bleeding and risk of infection. Prompt management is required to prevent complications. Complete abortion involves full expulsion with minimal bleeding. Threatened abortion presents with a closed cervix. ##

Q33. Answer: A

Explanation: Shock in pregnancy is most commonly associated with hemorrhage, especially in obstetric emergencies. Signs such as hypotension and tachycardia indicate circulatory compromise. Immediate fluid resuscitation is critical. Infection may also cause shock but usually includes fever. Rapid identification and treatment of bleeding are essential to prevent mortality. ##

Q34. Answer: B

Explanation: Fever with purulent vaginal discharge suggests pelvic or reproductive tract infection. This may involve the uterus or surrounding structures. It requires prompt antibiotic therapy to prevent spread. Other infections typically present with different primary symptoms. Early treatment reduces complications. ##

Q35. Answer: A

Explanation: Threatened abortion is characterized by light bleeding with a closed cervix and a viable pregnancy. The uterus size matches gestational age, indicating ongoing pregnancy. It may progress or resolve with monitoring. Incomplete abortion involves cervical dilation and tissue loss. Ectopic pregnancy presents with more severe symptoms. ##

Q36. Answer: C

Explanation: Molar pregnancy presents with heavy bleeding, enlarged uterus, and absence of a viable fetus. It involves abnormal trophoblastic proliferation. Additional signs may include excessive nausea and early complications. Diagnosis is confirmed with ultrasound and laboratory findings. Prompt management is necessary to prevent complications. ##

Q37. Answer: B

Explanation: Abdominal pain with rebound tenderness and fever suggests infection or intra-abdominal inflammation. This may involve uterine or pelvic structures. Prompt evaluation is required to identify the source. Hypertension and placenta previa do not present with these findings. Early intervention prevents progression to severe illness. ##

Q38. Answer: B

Explanation: Complete abortion occurs when all products of conception are expelled. Bleeding usually decreases afterward and the cervix closes. The uterus becomes smaller than expected for gestational age. Incomplete abortion involves retained tissue and continued bleeding. Proper assessment ensures no retained products remain. ##

Q39. Answer: D

Explanation: Ultrasound is essential in evaluating early pregnancy bleeding to determine viability and location. It helps diagnose conditions such as ectopic pregnancy or molar pregnancy. Other assessments provide supportive information but are not definitive. Early imaging allows timely and appropriate management. ##

Q40. Answer: A

Explanation: Foul-smelling discharge with systemic signs indicates infection that may progress to sepsis. This is a serious complication requiring immediate antibiotic therapy. Retained products can contribute to infection. Early recognition and treatment are critical. Other options do not present with infection signs. ##

Q41. Answer: B

Explanation: Ectopic pregnancy can present with abdominal pain, distension, and referred shoulder pain due to internal bleeding. These symptoms suggest possible rupture and hemoperitoneum. It is a life-threatening emergency requiring rapid diagnosis and intervention. Threatened abortion does not cause severe internal bleeding signs. Early recognition is essential to prevent maternal mortality. ##

Q42. Answer: B

Explanation: Heavy bleeding is defined as rapid saturation of a pad within minutes and passage of large clots. This indicates significant blood loss requiring urgent evaluation. It may be associated with complications like incomplete abortion. Light bleeding occurs more slowly and is less severe. Prompt management is needed to prevent shock. ##

Q43. Answer: A

Explanation: A uterus smaller than expected along with bleeding suggests complete abortion. This occurs when all products of conception are expelled. The uterus begins to involute after expulsion. Molar pregnancy typically presents with an enlarged uterus. Incomplete abortion would still have retained tissue. ##

Q44. Answer: A

Explanation: In suspected ectopic pregnancy, the structure is fragile and can rupture easily. A forceful bimanual exam may cause rupture leading to internal bleeding. Gentle examination reduces this risk. Although diagnosis is important, safety is the priority. Preventing rupture is critical to avoid life-threatening complications. ##

Q45. Answer: A

Explanation: Infection after abortion can progress to sepsis if not treated promptly. Symptoms include fever, malaise, and foul-smelling discharge. This indicates systemic infection that may worsen rapidly. Early antibiotic treatment is essential. Other conditions do not present with systemic infection signs. ##

Q46. Answer: A

Explanation: Shock without visible bleeding suggests possible internal hemorrhage. Conditions like ruptured ectopic pregnancy or concealed abruption should be considered. Internal bleeding can rapidly lead to hemodynamic instability. Immediate assessment and intervention are required. Delayed recognition increases risk of mortality. ##

Q47. Answer: B

Explanation: Threatened abortion is managed with observation and monitoring as pregnancy may continue. The cervix is closed and bleeding is usually mild. Immediate intervention is not required unless condition worsens. Surgical or medical treatment is not indicated initially. Regular follow-up ensures early detection of progression. ##

Q48. Answer: C

Explanation: Peritonitis indicates severe intra-abdominal infection and inflammation. Symptoms such as fever and abdominal pain with rigidity are concerning. It may result from uterine or bowel complications. Immediate intervention is required to prevent deterioration. Mild conditions do not present with such severe findings. ##

Q49. Answer: D

Explanation: Inevitable abortion is characterized by bleeding and cervical dilation without expulsion yet. The pregnancy cannot continue due to cervical opening. It typically progresses to incomplete or complete abortion. Threatened abortion has a closed cervix. Early identification helps guide appropriate management. ##

Q50. Answer: D

Explanation: Fetal heart rates below 100 or above 180 bpm indicate possible fetal distress. These abnormal values suggest compromised oxygenation. Prompt evaluation is required to determine cause and intervention. Normal baseline ranges from 110 to 160 bpm. Early detection helps prevent adverse outcomes. ##

Q51. Answer: C

Explanation: Shock is identified by hypotension, tachycardia, and altered mental status. These signs reflect inadequate tissue perfusion and oxygen delivery. In pregnancy, it is often related to hemorrhage or severe complications. Immediate management is required to stabilize circulation. Other options may cause some symptoms but do not fully explain this combination. ##

Q52. Answer: C

Explanation: Painful urination with fever suggests a urinary tract infection. This is a common cause of fever during pregnancy. It can progress if untreated and affect maternal health. Early diagnosis allows prompt antibiotic treatment. Other infections typically present with different primary symptoms. ##

Q53. Answer: A

Explanation: Severe abdominal tenderness with fever and respiratory changes suggests a serious infection. These signs may indicate peritonitis or intra-abdominal complications. Immediate evaluation is required to determine the cause. Normal pregnancy does not produce such severe findings. Early intervention prevents worsening of the condition. ##

Q54. Answer: C

Explanation: Cyanosis and respiratory distress indicate impaired oxygenation. This is a life-threatening condition requiring immediate attention. Assessment of airway and breathing is the first priority. Other factors are secondary to maintaining adequate oxygen supply. Prompt intervention improves survival outcomes. ##

Q55. Answer: D

Explanation: Blood-stained mucus discharge, known as "show," along with contractions indicates onset of labor. It reflects cervical changes and preparation for delivery. This is a normal physiological process when occurring at appropriate gestation. Infection would present with fever and other symptoms. Recognition helps guide appropriate care. ##

Q56. Answer: A

Explanation: Rupture of membranes with contractions suggests progression toward labor. Immediate assessment of labor progress is required. Monitoring helps determine stage and necessary interventions. Antibiotics are used only if infection risk is identified. Timely evaluation ensures safe management. ##

Q57. Answer: A

Explanation: Severe headache with visual disturbances suggests neurological involvement. This may be associated with hypertensive complications in pregnancy. It increases the risk of seizures and requires urgent evaluation. Gastrointestinal or muscular causes do not present with these combined findings. Early management prevents serious outcomes. ##

Q58. Answer: C

Explanation: Pallor, weakness, and fainting suggest anemia and reduced oxygen-carrying capacity. This condition affects both maternal and fetal health. Early detection allows appropriate treatment. Hypertension does not typically cause pallor. Management improves overall pregnancy outcomes. ##

Q59. Answer: C

Explanation: Uterine atony is a major cause of postpartum hemorrhage. The uterus fails to contract effectively, leading to excessive bleeding. Immediate intervention is required to control blood loss. Infection may contribute but is not the primary cause here. Prompt treatment reduces maternal risk. ##

Q60. Answer: A

Explanation: Fever with neck stiffness and altered consciousness suggests severe systemic infection. This may indicate central nervous system involvement. Immediate evaluation and treatment are necessary. Mild conditions do not present with such serious signs. Early intervention is critical to prevent complications. ##

Q61. Answer: D

Explanation: Early pregnancy with abdominal pain, bleeding, and signs of shock strongly suggests ectopic pregnancy. Hypotension and pallor indicate internal bleeding, which may result from rupture. This is a medical emergency requiring immediate intervention. Threatened abortion usually does not present with shock. Early diagnosis is critical to prevent maternal mortality. ##

Q62. Answer: B

Explanation: Inevitable abortion is characterized by heavy bleeding, cervical dilation, and cramping without expulsion yet. The pregnancy cannot continue due to cervical opening. It usually progresses to incomplete or complete abortion. Threatened abortion has a closed cervix. Early recognition guides timely management decisions. ##

Q63. Answer: D

Explanation: Post-abortion infection with systemic signs such as fever and foul discharge indicates possible sepsis. This condition can progress rapidly and become life-threatening. Immediate antibiotic therapy is essential. Mild infection would not present with severe systemic symptoms. Early intervention improves survival outcomes. ##

Q64. Answer: B

Explanation: Passage of tissue followed by reduced uterine size suggests complete abortion. The uterus contracts after expulsion of all products of conception. Bleeding typically decreases afterward. Incomplete abortion would show continued bleeding due to retained tissue. Proper assessment ensures no remaining complications. ##

Q65. Answer: B

Explanation: Rebound tenderness and rigid abdomen with fever indicate peritonitis. This is a severe intra-abdominal inflammatory condition. It may result from infection or organ rupture. Immediate evaluation and intervention are required. Mild conditions do not present with such severe findings. Early management prevents deterioration. ##

Q66. Answer: A

Explanation: Threatened abortion presents with bleeding and mild cramping but a closed cervix and viable pregnancy. The condition may resolve without progression. Close monitoring is required. Incomplete and inevitable abortion involve cervical dilation. Early identification helps guide appropriate care. ##

Q67. Answer: D

Explanation: Shock without external bleeding suggests concealed internal hemorrhage. Conditions like ruptured ectopic pregnancy or concealed abruption may cause this. Rapid assessment is necessary to identify the source. Delay in recognition increases mortality risk. Immediate intervention is critical. ##

Q68. Answer: C

Explanation: Signs of infection with purulent discharge require immediate antibiotic therapy. Delay in treatment can lead to worsening infection or sepsis. Observation alone is insufficient in this scenario. Early intervention helps control infection and prevent complications. Prompt management improves outcomes. ##

Q69. Answer: D

Explanation: Molar pregnancy presents with abnormal tissue growth, absence of a viable fetus, and enlarged uterus. It results from abnormal fertilization and trophoblastic proliferation. Bleeding is a common symptom. Diagnosis is confirmed with imaging findings. Early treatment is required to prevent complications. ##

Q70. Answer: D

Explanation: Incomplete abortion involves partial expulsion of products with continued bleeding. Retained tissue prevents uterine contraction and leads to hemorrhage. Immediate management is required to remove remaining tissue. Complete abortion would show minimal bleeding. Early intervention prevents complications such as infection. ##

Q71. Answer: C

Explanation: Cyanosis and respiratory distress indicate inadequate oxygenation. This is a critical condition requiring immediate airway and breathing assessment. Oxygen delivery must be prioritized to prevent tissue hypoxia. Cardiac and fluid issues may contribute but are secondary. Prompt intervention is essential for maternal survival. ##

Q72. Answer: C

Explanation: Fever with painful urination suggests urinary tract infection. This is a common cause of fever during pregnancy. If untreated, it may progress to more severe infection. Early diagnosis allows timely antibiotic therapy. Other infections present with different symptom patterns. ##

Q73. Answer: C

Explanation: Hypotension with tachycardia and abdominal pain indicates shock. This may result from internal bleeding or severe complications. Immediate assessment and fluid resuscitation are required. Delay in treatment increases mortality risk. Other conditions do not explain the severity of findings. ##

Q74. Answer: D

Explanation: Severe abdominal pain with rigidity and no visible bleeding suggests concealed hemorrhage. This may occur in conditions where blood accumulates internally. It can rapidly lead to shock if untreated. Immediate evaluation is required. Other options do not present with these findings. ##

Q75. Answer: B

Explanation: Signs of infection with foul discharge require immediate antibiotic therapy. Delay in treatment increases risk of sepsis. Observation alone is not appropriate in this scenario. Early management helps control infection and prevent complications. Prompt intervention improves maternal outcomes. ##

Q76. Answer: C

Explanation: Threatened abortion presents with mild bleeding and a closed cervix. The pregnancy may continue with proper monitoring. There is no expulsion of tissue. Other forms involve cervical dilation or tissue passage. Early identification helps guide observation and follow-up. ##

Q77. Answer: B

Explanation: Rebound tenderness and fever indicate peritonitis, a severe intra-abdominal infection. This condition can worsen rapidly without treatment. Immediate medical intervention is required. Mild conditions do not present with such severity. Early recognition is critical to prevent life-threatening outcomes. ##

Q78. Answer: C

Explanation: Incomplete abortion involves partial expulsion of tissue with continued bleeding. The cervix remains dilated and bleeding persists. Retained tissue prevents uterine contraction. Immediate management is required to control bleeding. Complete abortion would show cessation of bleeding. ##

Q79. Answer: B

Explanation: Molar pregnancy presents with enlarged uterus and absence of fetal heart activity. It involves abnormal tissue growth rather than a viable fetus. Bleeding is commonly present. Diagnosis is confirmed through imaging. Early management is necessary to prevent complications. ##

Q80. Answer: D

Explanation: After stabilizing a patient in shock, identifying the underlying cause is essential. This guides further management and treatment. Delaying diagnosis may worsen the condition. Discharge is inappropriate in unstable cases. A systematic approach improves outcomes and ensures proper care. ##

Q81. Answer: D

Explanation: Difficulty breathing with wheezing indicates involvement of the respiratory system. Pallor may suggest associated hypoxia or anemia. Immediate assessment of airway and breathing is essential. Cardiovascular causes may contribute but do not explain wheezing. Early management ensures adequate oxygen delivery and prevents complications. ##

Q82. Answer: B

Explanation: Cool clammy skin, hypotension, and weak pulse are classic signs of shock. These findings indicate poor tissue perfusion. Immediate fluid resuscitation and stabilization are required. Mild dehydration does not present with severe hypotension. Early intervention is critical to prevent deterioration. ##

Q83. Answer: D

Explanation: Failure of placenta delivery after childbirth suggests retained placenta. This can lead to significant bleeding and complications. Immediate management is necessary to prevent hemorrhage. Normal recovery would involve complete expulsion. Early recognition allows timely intervention. ##

Q84. Answer: A

Explanation: Fever with neck stiffness and altered breathing suggests severe infection. It may involve central nervous system or systemic spread. Immediate medical evaluation is required. Mild illnesses do not present with these findings. Early treatment helps prevent life-threatening complications. ##

Q85. Answer: B

Explanation: Signs of shock require immediate fluid resuscitation to restore circulation. This is the priority before diagnostic procedures. Delay in treatment can worsen outcomes. Oral medications are not appropriate in unstable patients. Early intervention stabilizes the patient and prevents complications. ##

Q86. Answer: A

Explanation: Fever with abdominal tenderness and purulent discharge suggests pelvic infection. This involves reproductive organs and requires prompt treatment. Delay may lead to systemic infection. Other infections present with different symptoms. Early antibiotic therapy is essential for recovery. ##

Q87. Answer: B

Explanation: Weakness, pallor, and fainting suggest anemia due to reduced oxygen-carrying capacity. This condition affects maternal and fetal health. Early identification allows treatment with supplementation. Hypertension does not cause pallor. Proper management improves outcomes. ##

Q88. Answer: A

Explanation: Determining gestational age and recent delivery helps identify the cause of bleeding. Different causes are associated with different stages of pregnancy. This information guides appropriate management. Other factors are less relevant in this context. Accurate assessment improves clinical decision-making. ##

Q89. Answer: C

Explanation: Severe pain with a rigid uterus and shock suggests placental abruption. This condition involves premature separation of the placenta. It can cause internal bleeding and fetal compromise. Immediate intervention is required. Placenta previa typically presents with painless bleeding. ##

Q90. Answer: D

Explanation: Symptoms of fever and painful urination indicate possible infection. Early evaluation helps confirm diagnosis and initiate treatment. Delay may lead to complications. Ignoring symptoms is unsafe. Prompt assessment ensures appropriate management. ##

Q91. Answer: B

Explanation: Cyanosis and shallow breathing indicate compromised oxygenation, requiring immediate assessment of airway and breathing. This is a life-threatening situation if not addressed promptly. Oxygen delivery must be ensured to maintain tissue perfusion. Other assessments can follow once stabilization occurs. Early intervention is essential to prevent deterioration. ##

Q92. Answer: D

Explanation: A fast weak pulse, cold clammy skin, and low blood pressure are hallmark signs of shock. These findings indicate poor circulation and inadequate perfusion. Immediate fluid resuscitation is required. Infection may cause fever but not all shock features. Early recognition improves survival outcomes. ##

Q93. Answer: A

Explanation: Fever with painful and frequent urination suggests urinary tract infection. This is a common condition during pregnancy. If untreated, it can lead to complications. Early diagnosis allows prompt antibiotic treatment. Other infections do not present with these urinary symptoms. ##

Q94. Answer: D

Explanation: Determining pregnancy status or recent childbirth helps identify the cause of vaginal bleeding. Different causes are associated with different stages. This information guides clinical decision-making. Other factors are not directly related to bleeding causes. Accurate history improves diagnosis and management. ##

Q95. Answer: C

Explanation: Severe abdominal pain with hypotension and tachycardia indicates shock. This may result from internal bleeding or other complications. Immediate stabilization is required. Mild discomfort does not present with such severe signs. Early intervention prevents further deterioration. ##

Q96. Answer: A

Explanation: Fever, tenderness, and purulent discharge indicate pelvic infection. This involves reproductive structures and requires prompt treatment. Delay may lead to systemic infection. Other conditions do not present with these findings. Early antibiotic therapy is essential. ##

Q97. Answer: A

Explanation: Pallor, weakness, and dizziness suggest anemia due to reduced hemoglobin levels. This affects oxygen delivery to tissues. Early identification allows appropriate treatment. Hypertension does not cause pallor. Proper management improves maternal and fetal outcomes. ##

Q98. Answer: B

Explanation: Uterine atony leads to failure of uterine contraction, causing hemorrhage. This is a major cause of postpartum bleeding. Immediate intervention is required to control blood loss. Infection may occur later but is not the primary issue. Early management prevents severe complications. ##

Q99. Answer: B

Explanation: Fever with neck stiffness and altered mental status suggests severe systemic or central nervous system infection. This is a life-threatening condition. Immediate medical evaluation is required. Mild illnesses do not present with these severe findings. Early treatment is critical for survival. ##

Q100. Answer: A

Explanation: Rapid assessment is essential in managing vaginal bleeding during pregnancy. Early evaluation helps determine severity and cause. Delayed assessment can worsen outcomes. Reassurance alone is insufficient in acute situations. Prompt action ensures timely and appropriate care. ## Question (101-200)

Question (101-200)

Q101. A pregnant woman undergoes a nonstress test that fails to show adequate accelerations within 20 minutes. What is this result called?

(A) Normal variation
(B) Inconclusive tracing
(C) Nonreactive pattern
(D) Reactive pattern

Q102. A pregnant patient at 30 weeks has a nonreactive NST. What is the most appropriate next step?

(A) Ignore findings
(B) Immediate delivery
(C) Discharge patient
(D) Perform additional testing

Q103. A pregnant woman is diagnosed with gestational hypertension. How is this condition classified?

(A) Neurological disorder
(B) Pregnancy-related new hypertension
(C) Chronic condition before pregnancy
(D) Infectious condition

Q104. A pregnant patient is identified as high risk for antepartum testing. Which condition is included as an indication?

(A) Normal weight gain
(B) Mild nausea
(C) Routine discomfort
(D) Decreased fetal movement

Q105. A pregnant woman has multiple gestation and is being monitored for complications. What risk is significantly increased?

(A) Post-term pregnancy
(B) Reduced uterine activity
(C) Preterm birth
(D) Decreased fetal demand

Q106. A pregnant patient has a history of previous preterm birth. What is her risk in the current pregnancy?

(A) Increased recurrence risk
(B) Reduced complication risk
(C) Unrelated to outcome
(D) No increased risk

Q107. A pregnant woman with substance abuse history is evaluated. What complication is associated with this factor?

(A) Preterm labor
(B) Post-term pregnancy
(C) Delayed labor onset
(D) Reduced fetal growth only

Q108. A pregnant patient presents with vaginal bleeding and uterine tenderness without fever. What diagnosis is most likely?

(A) Normal labor
(B) Placental abruption
(C) Urinary infection
(D) Placenta previa

Q109. A pregnant woman is evaluated for placental abruption. Which risk factor is commonly associated?
(A) Adequate hydration
(B) Low activity level
(C) Balanced diet
(D) Chronic hypertension
Q110. A pregnant patient is in early pregnancy phase where uterus remains relaxed and cervix is firm. What phase is this?
(A) Active labor phase
(B) Recovery phase
(C) Uterine quiescence
(D) Expulsion phase
Q111. A pregnant woman undergoes a biophysical profile showing reduced fetal breathing movements but normal fluid and tone. What does this indicate?
(A) No need for follow-up
(B) Possible fetal compromise
(C) Normal fetal condition
(D) Immediate fetal death
Q112. A pregnant patient has decreased fetal movement and is sent for antenatal testing. What is the primary purpose of such testing?
(A) Assess fetal well-being
(B) Measure maternal weight
(C) Evaluate uterine size
(D) Determine fetal gender
Q113. A pregnant woman at risk for preterm labor is being evaluated. Which factor increases her risk significantly?
(A) Previous preterm birth
(B) Normal BMI
(C) Regular exercise
(D) Adequate nutrition
Q114. A pregnant patient presents with painless vaginal bleeding during the third trimester. What is the most likely condition?
(A) Placental abruption
(B) Placenta previa
(C) Uterine rupture
(D) Infection
Q115. A pregnant woman is found to have moderate variability on fetal monitoring. What does this finding suggest?
(A) Immediate distress
(B) Normal fetal status
(C) Fetal hypoxia
(D) Neurological damage
Q116. A pregnant patient with hypertension develops seizures during pregnancy. What condition does this indicate?
(A) Preeclampsia
(B) Eclampsia
(C) Chronic hypertension
(D) Gestational hypertension

Q117. A pregnant woman is undergoing NST and shows two accelerations within 20 minutes. What is this result?
(A) Nonreactive test
(B) Reactive test
(C) Abnormal pattern
(D) Incomplete test
Q118. A pregnant patient presents with abdominal pain, uterine tenderness, and vaginal bleeding. What condition should be suspected?
(A) Normal labor
(B) Placenta previa
(C) Urinary infection
(D) Placental abruption
Q119. A pregnant woman is in the phase where the uterus becomes responsive to stimulants preparing for labor. What is this phase called?
(A) Expulsion phase
(B) Recovery phase
(C) Activation phase
(D) Uterine quiescence
Q120. A pregnant patient with diabetes is monitored for fetal well-being. Why is she considered high risk?
(A) Delayed fetal growth only
(B) Increased fetal oxygenation
(C) Reduced need for testing
(D) Risk of fetal compromise
Q121. A pregnant woman undergoes a biophysical profile and receives a low score. What does this result indicate?
(A) Possible fetal compromise
(B) Confirmed fetal death
(C) No clinical concern
(D) Normal fetal activity
Q122. A pregnant patient is advised antenatal testing due to chronic hypertension. What is the reason for this recommendation?
(A) Reduce maternal stress
(B) Increase fetal size
(C) Improve maternal nutrition
(D) Monitor fetal well-being
Q123. A pregnant woman reports sudden onset vaginal bleeding without pain in the third trimester. Which diagnosis is most likely?
(A) Placental abruption
(B) Infection
(C) Placenta previa
(D) Uterine rupture
Q124. A pregnant patient with a history of smoking is evaluated for preterm labor risk. What is the associated complication?
(A) Reduced uterine activity
(B) Delayed labor
(C) Preterm birth
(D) Post-term pregnancy

Q125. A pregnant woman undergoing NST shows normal accelerations and variability. What is the interpretation?
(A) Nonreactive pattern
(B) Incomplete result
(C) Reactive pattern
(D) Abnormal tracing
Q126. A pregnant patient presents with uterine tenderness, vaginal bleeding, and signs of distress. What condition is most likely?
(A) Urinary infection
(B) Placenta previa
(C) Placental abruption
(D) Normal labor
Q127. A pregnant woman is in the phase where hormonal changes increase uterine sensitivity to stimulation. What phase is this?
(A) Quiescent phase
(B) Recovery phase
(C) Activation phase
(D) Expulsion phase
Q128. A pregnant patient presents with decreased fetal movement and is scheduled for testing. Which test is commonly used initially?
(A) Blood test
(B) X-ray imaging
(C) Nonstress test
(D) Biophysical profile
Q129. A pregnant woman with diabetes is monitored regularly. What is the primary concern for the fetus?
(A) Increased growth only
(B) Reduced activity only
(C) Delayed labor only
(D) Compromised oxygenation
Q130. A pregnant patient develops seizures after diagnosis of preeclampsia. What condition does this progression represent?
(A) Mild hypertension
(B) Chronic hypertension
(C) Eclampsia
(D) Gestational hypertension
Q131. A pregnant woman undergoes NST and no accelerations are noted even after stimulation. What is the likely interpretation?
(A) Reactive result
(B) Nonreactive result
(C) Normal finding
(D) Reassuring pattern
Q132. A pregnant patient presents with bleeding and a soft non-tender uterus. What condition is most consistent?
(A) Placental abruption
(B) Placenta previa
(C) Preterm labor
(D) Infection

Q133. A pregnant woman is identified as high risk due to decreased fetal movement. What is the main goal of testing?
(A) Evaluate maternal weight
(B) Confirm fetal gender
(C) Assess fetal oxygenation
(D) Measure uterine size
Q134. A pregnant patient has multiple gestation and is monitored closely. What complication is commonly associated?
(A) Reduced contractions
(B) Post-term delivery
(C) Delayed labor
(D) Preterm birth
Q135. A pregnant woman is in early pregnancy where uterus remains inactive and cervix is firm. What phase is this?
(A) Recovery phase
(B) Quiescent phase
(C) Activation phase
(D) Expulsion phase
Q136. A pregnant patient presents with uterine tenderness and vaginal bleeding with signs of distress. What is the likely diagnosis?
(A) Normal labor
(B) Placenta previa
(C) Placental abruption
(D) Urinary infection
Q137. A pregnant woman undergoes antenatal testing and shows reassuring results. What does this indicate?
(A) Immediate delivery needed
(B) Normal fetal status
(C) Abnormal condition
(D) Fetal compromise
Q138. A pregnant patient with hypertension is monitored regularly. What is the main fetal risk?
(A) Oxygen compromise
(B) Increased activity
(C) Excess growth
(D) Delayed movement
Q139. A pregnant woman shows moderate variability on fetal monitoring. What does this indicate?
(A) Normal function
(B) Acidosis
(C) Fetal distress
(D) Hypoxia
Q140. A pregnant patient presents with vaginal bleeding and uterine pain. What is the most likely condition?
(A) Normal change
(B) Placental abruption
(C) Infection
(D) Placenta previa
Q141. A pregnant woman undergoes NST with normal findings. What does this suggest about fetal status?

(A) Reassuring
(B) Inconclusive
(C) Compromised
(D) Abnormal

Q142. A pregnant patient has decreased fetal movement and abnormal NST. What is the next step?
(A) Discharge patient
(B) Perform further testing
(C) Delay evaluation
(D) Ignore findings

Q143. A pregnant woman presents with risk factors including smoking and previous preterm birth. What complication is most likely?
(A) Reduced contractions
(B) Post-term pregnancy
(C) Delayed delivery
(D) Preterm labor

Q144. A pregnant patient is evaluated for placental abruption. Which symptom supports this diagnosis?
(A) No bleeding
(B) Uterine tenderness
(C) Soft uterus
(D) Painless bleeding

Q145. A pregnant woman is in the phase preparing uterus for labor through hormonal changes. What is this phase?
(A) Quiescent phase
(B) Recovery phase
(C) Activation phase
(D) Expulsion phase

Q146. A pregnant patient presents with abnormal NST findings. What is the main concern?
(A) Nutritional issue
(B) Maternal stress
(C) Fetal compromise
(D) Normal variation

Q147. A pregnant woman undergoes BPP and receives normal results. What does this indicate?
(A) Adequate oxygenation
(B) Abnormal condition
(C) Compromised fetus
(D) Immediate delivery needed

Q148. A pregnant patient presents with vaginal bleeding and uterine rigidity. What is the most likely diagnosis?
(A) Normal contraction
(B) Placenta previa
(C) Infection
(D) Placental abruption

Q149. A pregnant woman is monitored for decreased fetal movement. What is the initial assessment tool?
(A) Imaging study
(B) Biophysical profile
(C) Blood test

(D) Nonstress test

Q150. A pregnant patient with hypertension is undergoing antenatal testing. What is the purpose of this monitoring?

(A) Detect fetal compromise

(B) Improve maternal nutrition

(C) Reduce contractions

(D) Increase fetal growth

Q151. Gestational diabetes increases the risk of which maternal complication?

(A) Delayed fetal movement

(B) Development of preeclampsia

(C) Reduced uterine tone

(D) Decreased blood glucose

Q152. Screening for gestational diabetes is commonly performed during which gestational period?

(A) 24-28 weeks

(B) 16-18 weeks

(C) 32-34 weeks

(D) 10-12 weeks

Q153. A pregnant woman with elevated glucose levels is at risk of delivering an infant with increased birth weight. What is this condition called?

(A) Growth restriction

(B) Microcephaly

(C) Hypotrophy

(D) Macrosomia

Q154. Gestational diabetes is associated with an increased long-term risk of which condition in the mother?

(A) Thyroid disorder

(B) Type 2 diabetes

(C) Type 1 diabetes

(D) Cardiac anomaly

Q155. A pregnant woman undergoes a glucose challenge test and has elevated results. What is the next step?

(A) Repeat test after delivery

(B) Immediate insulin therapy

(C) Discharge patient

(D) Perform glucose tolerance test

Q156. A pregnant patient with gestational diabetes presents with excessive amniotic fluid. What condition is this?

(A) Amniotic rupture

(B) Polyhydramnios

(C) Oligohydramnios

(D) Normal fluid volume

Q157. A pregnant woman with gestational diabetes delivers a newborn who develops low blood sugar shortly after birth. What is the likely cause?

(A) Maternal hypoglycemia

(B) Reduced placental flow

(C) Delayed feeding

(D) Fetal hyperinsulinemia

Q158. A pregnant patient is being screened early due to risk factors for diabetes. What is the purpose of early screening?
(A) Detect fetal anomalies
(B) Measure fetal weight
(C) Identify preexisting diabetes
(D) Assess uterine size
Q159. A pregnant woman is diagnosed with gestational diabetes after confirmatory testing. What is the primary goal of management?
(A) Reduce maternal weight
(B) Maintain normal glucose levels
(C) Increase fetal growth
(D) Delay labor onset
Q160. A pregnant patient with poorly controlled diabetes presents with excessive fetal growth and increased amniotic fluid on ultrasound. What complication is most likely developing?
(A) Growth restriction
(B) Delayed labor progression
(C) Macrosomia with polyhydramnios
(D) Reduced fetal activity
Q161. Gestational diabetes increases the risk of which neonatal complication?
(A) Hyperbilirubinemia
(B) Delayed reflexes
(C) Decreased tone
(D) Reduced activity
Q162. A one-hour glucose screening test uses which glucose amount?
(A) 50-gram load
(B) 25-gram load
(C) 75-gram load
(D) 100-gram load
Q163. A pregnant woman with uncontrolled diabetes is at risk for which delivery complication?
(A) Shoulder dystocia
(B) Delayed cervical dilation
(C) Reduced contractions
(D) Prolonged quiescence
Q164. Universal screening for gestational diabetes is recommended because many women have risk factors.
(A) Not clinically relevant
(B) True statement
(C) False statement
(D) Depends on trimester
Q165. A pregnant patient undergoes a 3-hour glucose tolerance test after abnormal screening. What is the purpose of this test?
(A) Confirm diagnosis
(B) Monitor fetal growth
(C) Evaluate placental size
(D) Assess uterine activity
Q166. A pregnant woman with gestational diabetes presents with excessive fetal growth and is being monitored closely. What is the primary concern during delivery?
(A) Reduced contractions

(B) Shoulder dystocia
(C) Delayed labor
(D) Preterm rupture

Q167. A pregnant patient with gestational diabetes is counseled about long-term health risks. What should be included in teaching?

(A) Risk of anemia only
(B) Risk of type 2 diabetes
(C) Risk of infection only
(D) Risk of thyroid disease

Q168. A pregnant woman presents at 26 weeks for routine care and undergoes glucose screening. Why is this timing appropriate?

(A) Peak fetal growth
(B) Reduced hormone levels
(C) Increased insulin resistance
(D) Decreased blood volume

Q169. A pregnant patient with gestational diabetes has elevated glucose levels despite diet control. What is the next step?

(A) Delay treatment
(B) Discharge patient
(C) Stop monitoring
(D) Initiate medication

Q170. A pregnant woman with gestational diabetes presents with excessive amniotic fluid, large fetus, and difficulty breathing. What is the most likely combined condition?

(A) Reduced fetal activity
(B) Normal pregnancy changes
(C) Polyhydramnios with macrosomia
(D) Oligohydramnios with restriction

Q171. Polyhydramnios in pregnancy is commonly associated with which maternal condition?

(A) Mild infection
(B) Nutritional deficiency
(C) Gestational diabetes
(D) Chronic anemia

Q172. A fetus exposed to high maternal glucose develops increased insulin production. What is this effect called?

(A) Glucose intolerance
(B) Insulin resistance
(C) Hypoinsulinemia
(D) Hyperinsulinemia

Q173. A large fetus due to maternal diabetes increases the risk of which birth complication?

(A) Preterm rupture
(B) Shoulder dystocia
(C) Reduced contractions
(D) Cervical insufficiency

Q174. Women with gestational diabetes should receive postpartum follow-up for which reason?

(A) Detect type 2 diabetes
(B) Evaluate nutrition
(C) Assess infection risk
(D) Monitor anemia

Q175. A pregnant patient has an abnormal glucose screening result. What diagnostic test is performed next?
(A) Hemoglobin level
(B) Urine glucose test
(C) Glucose tolerance test
(D) Random glucose test
Q176. A pregnant woman with gestational diabetes reports adherence to diet but still has elevated glucose levels. What is the appropriate management?
(A) Initiate pharmacologic therapy
(B) Delay further action
(C) Discontinue monitoring
(D) Continue diet only
Q177. A pregnant patient presents with excessive amniotic fluid and large fetal size during ultrasound evaluation. What underlying condition should be considered?
(A) Gestational diabetes
(B) Chronic hypertension
(C) Nutritional deficiency
(D) Mild infection
Q178. A pregnant woman is counseled regarding fetal risks associated with diabetes. Which complication should be emphasized?
(A) Macrosomia
(B) Reduced movement
(C) Growth restriction
(D) Delayed reflexes
Q179. A pregnant patient with diabetes has a fetus producing high insulin levels. What neonatal issue is most likely after birth?
(A) Hypoglycemia
(B) Hyperthermia
(C) Hyperglycemia
(D) Hypercalcemia
Q180. A pregnant woman with poorly controlled diabetes presents with shortness of breath, abdominal distension, and ultrasound showing excess fluid and large fetus. What is the most likely explanation for her condition?
(A) Polyhydramnios with macrosomia
(B) Normal pregnancy changes
(C) Oligohydramnios with restriction
(D) Reduced fetal activity
Q181. Fetal hyperinsulinemia primarily results from which maternal condition?
(A) Gestational diabetes
(B) Chronic anemia
(C) Mild infection
(D) Nutritional deficiency
Q182. The standard confirmatory test for gestational diabetes measures glucose over what duration?
(A) 3 hours
(B) 2 hours
(C) 4 hours
(D) 1 hour

Q183. A fetus exposed to persistent high glucose levels may develop excessive growth. What is the primary mechanism?
(A) Increased insulin secretion
(B) Decreased metabolism
(C) Reduced nutrient supply
(D) Impaired circulation
Q184. Which maternal condition increases the likelihood of polyhydramnios due to fetal osmotic diuresis?
(A) Gestational diabetes
(B) Chronic infection
(C) Nutritional imbalance
(D) Mild anemia
Q185. A pregnant woman with gestational diabetes has persistent elevated glucose despite diet control. What is the best next step?
(A) Repeat screening only
(B) Delay intervention
(C) Initiate medication therapy
(D) Stop dietary control
Q186. A pregnant patient with diabetes is being monitored for fetal complications. Which finding indicates increased risk during delivery?
(A) Small fetal size
(B) Large fetal size
(C) Reduced amniotic fluid
(D) Normal fetal tone
Q187. A pregnant woman presents with excessive amniotic fluid and is found to have gestational diabetes. What fetal process contributes to this finding?
(A) Impaired growth
(B) Increased urination
(C) Reduced urination
(D) Decreased circulation
Q188. A pregnant patient is counseled on neonatal risks related to maternal diabetes. Which condition commonly occurs after birth?
(A) Hypertension
(B) Hypoglycemia
(C) Hyperglycemia
(D) Hyperthermia
Q189. A pregnant woman undergoes testing due to risk factors and is diagnosed with gestational diabetes. What is the primary focus of treatment?
(A) Maintain normal glucose
(B) Delay labor
(C) Increase fetal growth
(D) Reduce uterine activity
Q190. A pregnant woman with poorly controlled diabetes presents with breathing discomfort, abdominal distension, and ultrasound findings of excess fluid and large fetus. What is the most likely underlying condition?
(A) Polyhydramnios with macrosomia
(B) Reduced fetal activity
(C) Growth restriction

(D) Normal adaptation

Q191. Excess fetal growth in diabetic pregnancy is primarily termed what?

(A) Growth delay
(B) Macrosomia
(C) Hypotrophy
(D) Microcephaly

Q192. The initial screening for gestational diabetes involves which type of test?

(A) Glucose challenge test
(B) Glucose tolerance test
(C) Random blood test
(D) Urine glucose test

Q193. A fetus exposed to high glucose levels develops increased fat deposition due to which hormone?

(A) Cortisol
(B) Glucagon
(C) Thyroxine
(D) Insulin

Q194. Polyhydramnios results from which fetal response in diabetic pregnancy?

(A) Increased urination
(B) Decreased circulation
(C) Reduced swallowing
(D) Impaired growth

Q195. A pregnant woman with gestational diabetes has persistently elevated glucose levels despite diet therapy. What is the next step in management?

(A) Discontinue monitoring
(B) Continue observation only
(C) Repeat screening later
(D) Initiate pharmacologic treatment

Q196. A pregnant patient with diabetes is being evaluated before delivery. Which finding increases the risk of delivery complications?

(A) Stable glucose levels
(B) Normal fluid level
(C) Reduced fetal weight
(D) Increased fetal size

Q197. A pregnant woman with gestational diabetes presents with excessive amniotic fluid. What mechanism explains this finding?

(A) Decreased maternal glucose
(B) Reduced fetal circulation
(C) Impaired placental flow
(D) Increased fetal urination

Q198. A pregnant patient with diabetes is counseled regarding neonatal complications. Which issue is most likely immediately after birth?

(A) Hypoglycemia
(B) Hyperthermia
(C) Hypertension
(D) Hyperglycemia

Q199. A pregnant woman diagnosed with gestational diabetes is advised on treatment goals. What is the primary objective?

(A) Maintain normal glucose levels
(B) Reduce uterine activity
(C) Increase fetal growth
(D) Delay labor onset

Q200. A pregnant woman with poorly controlled diabetes presents with breathing discomfort, abdominal enlargement, and ultrasound showing excess fluid and a large fetus. What is the most likely combined condition causing these findings?

(A) Reduced fetal activity
(B) Growth restriction pattern
(C) Normal physiological change
(D) Polyhydramnios with macrosomia

Answer Key and Explanation (101-200)

Q101. Answer: C

Explanation: A nonreactive NST is defined as failure to demonstrate sufficient fetal heart rate accelerations within a 20-minute period. This may occur due to fetal sleep, immaturity, or hypoxia. It does not immediately confirm fetal compromise but requires further evaluation. Additional testing such as BPP may be indicated. Reactive NST requires at least two accelerations. ##

Q102. Answer: D

Explanation: When NST is nonreactive, further assessment is required before discharge. This may include prolonging the test or performing a biophysical profile. Nonreactivity may be due to fetal sleep or immaturity. Immediate delivery is not indicated without further evaluation. Additional testing ensures accurate assessment of fetal well-being. ##

Q103. Answer: B

Explanation: Gestational hypertension refers to new-onset hypertension during pregnancy. It is part of the classification of hypertensive disorders specific to pregnancy. It differs from chronic hypertension which occurs before pregnancy. It must be monitored closely as it may progress. Proper classification guides management decisions. ##

Q104. Answer: D

Explanation: Decreased fetal movement is a key indication for antepartum fetal testing. It may signal compromised fetal well-being. Conditions like hypertension and diabetes are also included. Mild symptoms such as nausea are not indications. Early evaluation helps prevent adverse outcomes. ##

Q105. Answer: C

Explanation: Multiple gestation is a major risk factor for preterm birth. Uterine overdistension contributes to early contractions. Approximately 10% of preterm births are linked to multiple gestation. Close monitoring is required throughout pregnancy. Early intervention helps improve neonatal outcomes. ##

Q106. Answer: A

Explanation: Previous preterm birth significantly increases the risk of recurrence. The likelihood ranges from 20% to 40%. Risk varies depending on obstetric history. Careful monitoring is required in subsequent pregnancies. Early interventions may reduce recurrence risk. ##

Q107. Answer: A

Explanation: Substance abuse, including drugs and alcohol, is a known risk factor for preterm labor. It affects placental function and fetal environment. It may also lead to other complications. Early identification allows intervention and counseling. Prevention strategies improve pregnancy outcomes. ##

Q108. Answer: B

Explanation: Placental abruption presents with vaginal bleeding and uterine tenderness. It may occur without fever. It involves premature separation of the placenta. Risk factors include hypertension and trauma. Immediate assessment is required to prevent complications. ##

Q109. Answer: D

Explanation: Chronic hypertension is a significant risk factor for placental abruption. It contributes to vascular changes in the placenta. Other factors include trauma and substance use. Identification of risk factors helps in prevention and monitoring. Proper care reduces maternal and fetal risks. ##

Q110. Answer: C

Explanation: Uterine quiescence is the phase where the uterus remains relaxed and unresponsive. The cervix maintains structural integrity during this time. This phase represents most of pregnancy. It prevents premature contractions and delivery. Transition from this phase prepares for labor. ##

Q111. Answer: B

Explanation: A biophysical profile evaluates multiple parameters of fetal well-being. Reduction in fetal breathing movements may indicate early compromise. Other normal parameters may delay immediate intervention but require monitoring. It does not confirm fetal demise. Follow-up testing is essential to ensure continued fetal health. ##

Q112. Answer: A

Explanation: Antenatal testing is primarily used to assess fetal well-being and oxygenation. It helps identify fetuses at risk of hypoxia. Techniques include NST and BPP. Early detection allows timely intervention. Other options are not the purpose of these tests. ##

Q113. Answer: A

Explanation: Previous preterm birth is one of the strongest predictors of recurrence. The risk increases significantly compared to the general population. Monitoring is required in subsequent pregnancies. Preventive strategies may be applied. Other factors listed are not associated with increased risk. ##

Q114. Answer: B

Explanation: Placenta previa typically presents with painless vaginal bleeding. The placenta is located near or over the cervical opening. Unlike abruption, pain is usually absent. Diagnosis is confirmed with imaging. Management depends on severity and gestational age. ##

Q115. Answer: B

Explanation: Moderate variability reflects intact fetal autonomic function and adequate oxygenation. It is considered a reassuring sign. Absent or minimal variability may indicate compromise. Continuous monitoring helps detect changes. This finding supports normal fetal status. ##

Q116. Answer: B

Explanation: Eclampsia is defined as the occurrence of seizures in a patient with preeclampsia. It represents severe progression of hypertensive disorder. Immediate management is required to protect mother and fetus. Gestational hypertension does not involve seizures. Early detection of preeclampsia can prevent this complication. ##

Q117. Answer: B

Explanation: A reactive NST is defined by at least two accelerations within 20 minutes. This indicates good fetal oxygenation and neurological function. It is considered reassuring. Nonreactive tests lack these accelerations. No further testing is usually required if reactive. ##

Q118. Answer: D

Explanation: Placental abruption presents with pain, tenderness, and bleeding. It involves premature separation of the placenta. This can compromise fetal oxygenation. Immediate evaluation is required. Placenta previa typically presents without pain. ##

Q119. Answer: C

Explanation: The activation phase prepares the uterus for labor by increasing responsiveness. Hormonal changes promote uterine contractions. This phase follows uterine quiescence. It leads to the onset of labor. Proper progression ensures effective delivery process. ##

Q120. Answer: D

Explanation: Diabetes increases the risk of fetal compromise due to metabolic effects. It may affect placental function and fetal growth. Such patients require regular antenatal testing. Early detection helps prevent complications. Monitoring improves maternal and fetal outcomes. ##

Q121. Answer: A

Explanation: A low biophysical profile score suggests possible fetal compromise and inadequate oxygenation. It evaluates parameters such as movement, tone, breathing, and amniotic fluid. A reduced score requires further evaluation or intervention. It does not immediately confirm fetal death. Close monitoring is necessary to determine next steps. ##

Q122. Answer: D

Explanation: Chronic hypertension places the fetus at risk for compromised oxygenation. Antenatal testing helps monitor fetal status and detect early signs of distress. This allows timely intervention if needed. It does not directly affect maternal nutrition or fetal size. Regular assessment improves outcomes. ##

Q123. Answer: C

Explanation: Painless vaginal bleeding in late pregnancy is characteristic of placenta previa. The placenta covers or lies near the cervical opening. This leads to bleeding without uterine tenderness. Abruption usually involves pain. Diagnosis is confirmed through imaging and guides management. ##

Q124. Answer: C

Explanation: Smoking is a known risk factor for preterm labor and birth. It affects placental function and fetal development. This increases the likelihood of early delivery. Preventive counseling is important. Other options are not associated with smoking risk. ##

Q125. Answer: C

Explanation: Presence of accelerations and normal variability indicates a reactive NST. This suggests adequate fetal oxygenation and neurological function. It is considered reassuring. Nonreactive patterns lack these findings. No further immediate testing is required in reactive cases. ##

Q126. Answer: C

Explanation: Placental abruption presents with uterine tenderness and bleeding. It involves premature separation of the placenta. This condition can compromise fetal oxygenation. Immediate evaluation is required. Placenta previa typically presents without pain. ##

Q127. Answer: C

Explanation: The activation phase prepares the uterus for labor by increasing responsiveness. Hormonal influences enhance contractility. This phase follows uterine quiescence. It leads toward the onset of labor. Proper progression ensures effective labor process. ##

Q128. Answer: C

Explanation: The nonstress test is commonly used as the initial assessment for decreased fetal movement. It evaluates fetal heart rate response to movement. It is noninvasive and widely available. If results are abnormal, further testing such as BPP may be done. Early evaluation helps detect compromise. ##

Q129. Answer: D

Explanation: Diabetes in pregnancy can affect placental function and fetal oxygenation. This increases risk of fetal compromise. Regular monitoring helps detect abnormalities early. It is not limited to growth changes alone. Early intervention improves fetal outcomes. ##

Q130. Answer: C

Explanation: Eclampsia is the progression of preeclampsia with the occurrence of seizures. It represents a severe complication requiring immediate intervention. This condition threatens both maternal and fetal life. Early recognition and management are critical. Other hypertensive states do not include seizures. ##

Q131. Answer: B

Explanation: Absence of accelerations despite stimulation indicates a nonreactive NST. This may suggest fetal sleep or compromise. Further evaluation is required to determine fetal status. It is not considered reassuring. Additional testing ensures accurate assessment. ##

Q132. Answer: B

Explanation: Placenta previa presents with bleeding and a soft, non-tender uterus. Pain is typically absent. This differentiates it from placental abruption. Diagnosis is confirmed with imaging. Management depends on severity and gestational age. ##

Q133. Answer: C

Explanation: Decreased fetal movement may indicate reduced oxygenation. Testing aims to assess fetal well-being. Early detection allows timely intervention. Other parameters are not the primary goal. Proper monitoring improves outcomes. ##

Q134. Answer: D

Explanation: Multiple gestation increases risk of preterm birth due to uterine overdistension. This leads to early onset of contractions. Close monitoring is required. Other options are not commonly associated. Early intervention improves neonatal outcomes. ##

Q135. Answer: B

Explanation: The quiescent phase is characterized by uterine inactivity and cervical firmness. It maintains pregnancy during early stages. Hormonal influences suppress contractions. This phase continues until activation begins. It prevents premature labor. ##

Q136. Answer: C

Explanation: Placental abruption involves uterine tenderness and bleeding. It results from premature placental separation. This can compromise fetal oxygenation. Immediate evaluation is required. Placenta previa usually lacks tenderness. ##

Q137. Answer: B

Explanation: Reassuring results indicate adequate fetal oxygenation and well-being. No immediate intervention is required. Continued routine monitoring is appropriate. It does not indicate compromise. These findings support ongoing pregnancy management. ##

Q138. Answer: A

Explanation: Hypertension affects placental blood flow, leading to reduced oxygen delivery. This increases risk of fetal compromise. Monitoring helps detect early changes. It is not limited to activity or growth changes. Early intervention improves outcomes. ##

Q139. Answer: A

Explanation: Moderate variability indicates intact fetal autonomic function. It reflects good oxygenation and neurological status. This is a reassuring sign. Abnormal variability may suggest compromise. Continuous monitoring ensures timely detection of changes. ##

Q140. Answer: B

Explanation: Vaginal bleeding with uterine pain is characteristic of placental abruption. It involves premature placental separation. This condition requires urgent evaluation. Placenta previa typically presents without pain. Early management is critical. ##

Q141. Answer: A

Explanation: Normal NST findings indicate reassuring fetal status. Adequate accelerations and variability reflect good oxygenation. No immediate intervention is needed. Compromised fetuses show abnormal patterns. Continued monitoring ensures safety. ##

Q142. Answer: B

Explanation: Abnormal NST requires further evaluation such as BPP. This helps assess fetal condition more comprehensively. Ignoring findings may delay intervention. Early assessment prevents complications. Proper follow-up ensures accurate diagnosis. ##

Q143. Answer: D

Explanation: Smoking and previous preterm birth significantly increase risk of preterm labor. These factors affect uterine and placental function. Close monitoring is required. Preventive strategies may reduce risk. Early detection improves outcomes. ##

Q144. Answer: B

Explanation: Uterine tenderness is a key feature of placental abruption. It differentiates it from placenta previa. Pain is usually present. Early recognition is important for management. Immediate evaluation prevents complications. ##

Q145. Answer: C

Explanation: Activation phase prepares uterus for labor by increasing responsiveness. Hormonal changes enhance contractility. This phase follows quiescence. It leads to effective labor onset. Proper progression ensures delivery readiness. ##

Q146. Answer: C

Explanation: Abnormal NST findings suggest possible fetal compromise. It indicates potential inadequate oxygenation. Further evaluation is required. It is not considered normal variation. Early intervention improves fetal outcomes. ##

Q147. Answer: A

Explanation: Normal BPP indicates adequate fetal oxygenation and well-being. All parameters are within normal limits. No immediate intervention is required. Compromised fetuses show low scores. Continued monitoring ensures ongoing health. ##

Q148. Answer: D

Explanation: Uterine rigidity with bleeding suggests placental abruption. It involves premature placental separation. This can compromise fetal oxygenation. Immediate evaluation is necessary. Placenta previa usually lacks rigidity. ##

Q149. Answer: D

Explanation: Nonstress test is the first-line assessment for decreased fetal movement. It evaluates fetal heart rate response. It is noninvasive and widely used. Abnormal results require further testing. Early assessment improves outcomes. ##

Q150. Answer: A

Explanation: Hypertension can affect placental blood flow and fetal oxygenation. Antenatal testing helps detect early signs of compromise. This allows timely intervention. It does not directly affect growth or nutrition. Monitoring improves pregnancy outcomes. ##

Q151. Answer: B

Explanation: Gestational diabetes is associated with an increased risk of developing preeclampsia. Elevated glucose levels affect vascular function and placental health. This creates conditions that predispose to hypertensive disorders. Other options do not align with known complications. Monitoring helps reduce associated risks. ##

Q152. Answer: A

Explanation: Screening for gestational diabetes is recommended between 24 and 28 weeks of pregnancy. This timing corresponds with increased insulin resistance. Early screening may occur if risk factors are present. Routine screening at this stage helps detect cases effectively. Proper diagnosis guides management strategies. ##

Q153. Answer: D

Explanation: Macrosomia refers to excessive fetal growth often seen in pregnancies complicated by diabetes. High maternal glucose levels lead to increased fetal insulin production. This promotes growth and fat deposition. Other options represent reduced or abnormal growth patterns. Monitoring glucose levels reduces this risk. ##

Q154. Answer: B

Explanation: Women with gestational diabetes have a significantly increased risk of developing type 2 diabetes later in life. Studies show a large percentage develop it within decades. This highlights the importance of long-term follow-up. Lifestyle modifications may reduce this risk. Other conditions are not directly linked. ##

Q155. Answer: D

Explanation: An elevated glucose challenge test requires confirmation with a glucose tolerance test. This provides a definitive diagnosis of gestational diabetes. Immediate insulin is not started without confirmation. Delaying testing is inappropriate. Accurate diagnosis ensures proper management. ##

Q156. Answer: B

Explanation: Polyhydramnios refers to excessive amniotic fluid and is associated with gestational diabetes. Elevated glucose levels affect fetal urination and fluid balance. This condition increases risk of complications. Monitoring fluid levels is important. Other options do not describe increased fluid volume. ##

Q157. Answer: D

Explanation: Infants of diabetic mothers often develop hypoglycemia due to high insulin levels. During pregnancy, excess glucose stimulates fetal insulin production. After birth, glucose supply drops but insulin remains high. This leads to low blood sugar. Early feeding and monitoring are essential. ##

Q158. Answer: C

Explanation: Early screening aims to detect undiagnosed preexisting diabetes or prediabetes. This allows early management to reduce complications. It differs from routine screening later in pregnancy. Early identification improves maternal and fetal outcomes. Other options are unrelated to screening purpose. ##

Q159. Answer: B

Explanation: The primary goal in managing gestational diabetes is maintaining normal blood glucose levels. This reduces risks for both mother and fetus. Proper control prevents complications such as macrosomia and preeclampsia. Other options are not primary goals. Monitoring and treatment ensure better outcomes. ##

Q160. Answer: C

Explanation: Poorly controlled diabetes leads to fetal hyperglycemia and hyperinsulinemia, causing macrosomia. It also contributes to polyhydramnios due to increased fetal urination. These combined findings indicate metabolic imbalance. Early management is necessary to prevent delivery complications. Monitoring improves outcomes. ##

Q161. Answer: A

Explanation: Gestational diabetes increases the risk of neonatal hyperbilirubinemia. Elevated maternal glucose affects fetal metabolism and liver function. This leads to increased bilirubin production after birth. Early monitoring helps detect and manage this condition. Other options are not primary complications linked to maternal diabetes. ##

Q162. Answer: A

Explanation: The initial screening test for gestational diabetes involves a 50-gram glucose load. Blood glucose is measured one hour after ingestion. This is part of the two-step screening approach. Elevated results require further testing. Other glucose loads are used in different testing protocols. ##

Q163. Answer: A

Explanation: Macrosomia due to maternal diabetes increases the risk of shoulder dystocia during delivery. Excess fetal size makes passage through the birth canal difficult. This can lead to complications for both mother and infant. Proper glucose control reduces this risk. Other options are not directly associated. ##

Q164. Answer: B

Explanation: Universal screening is recommended because a large proportion of women have at least one risk factor. Risk-based screening may miss many cases. Universal testing ensures broader detection. Early identification improves outcomes. This approach is supported by major guidelines. ##

Q165. Answer: A

Explanation: The 3-hour glucose tolerance test confirms the diagnosis of gestational diabetes. It measures glucose levels over time after ingestion. This provides definitive diagnostic criteria. Screening tests alone are not sufficient. Accurate diagnosis guides management decisions. ##

Q166. Answer: B

Explanation: Excessive fetal growth increases the risk of shoulder dystocia during delivery. This complication can lead to birth injuries. Monitoring fetal size helps plan delivery approach. Proper glucose control reduces risk. Other options are less directly related to macrosomia. ##

Q167. Answer: B

Explanation: Women with gestational diabetes have a significant long-term risk of developing type 2 diabetes. This risk persists years after pregnancy. Counseling should include lifestyle modification and follow-up screening. Early prevention strategies are important. Other options are not primary long-term risks. ##

Q168. Answer: C

Explanation: Screening at 24-28 weeks is recommended due to increased insulin resistance during this period. Hormonal changes affect glucose metabolism. This timing helps detect gestational diabetes effectively. Earlier screening may miss cases. Proper timing ensures accurate diagnosis. ##

Q169. Answer: D

Explanation: If diet alone does not control glucose levels, medication is required to maintain euglycemia. This prevents complications such as macrosomia. Continuous monitoring guides treatment adjustments. Delaying treatment increases risk. Proper management improves outcomes. ##

Q170. Answer: C

Explanation: Gestational diabetes can lead to polyhydramnios and macrosomia simultaneously. Increased fetal urination contributes to excess fluid. Large fetal size may cause maternal discomfort. These findings indicate poor glucose control. Close monitoring and management are required to reduce complications. ##

Q171. Answer: C

Explanation: Polyhydramnios is commonly associated with gestational diabetes due to increased fetal urination. Elevated maternal glucose leads to fetal hyperglycemia and osmotic diuresis. This increases amniotic fluid volume. Other listed conditions are not strongly linked to this finding. Monitoring helps manage associated risks. ##

Q172. Answer: D

Explanation: Fetal hyperinsulinemia occurs in response to elevated maternal glucose levels. The fetus produces excess insulin to manage increased glucose. This contributes to macrosomia and metabolic complications. It is a key mechanism in diabetic pregnancies. Other options do not describe increased insulin levels. ##

Q173. Answer: B

Explanation: Macrosomia significantly increases the risk of shoulder dystocia during delivery. The large fetal size can obstruct passage through the birth canal. This may result in injury if not managed properly. Early identification helps plan delivery approach. Other options are less directly related. ##

Q174. Answer: A

Explanation: Gestational diabetes increases the long-term risk of type 2 diabetes. Postpartum follow-up is essential to detect early development. Lifestyle modifications can reduce this risk. Regular screening is recommended. Other options are not primary reasons for follow-up. ##

Q175. Answer: C

Explanation: After an abnormal screening, a glucose tolerance test is performed for confirmation. It measures blood glucose over time after ingestion. This test provides definitive diagnostic criteria. Screening alone is insufficient for diagnosis. Accurate testing guides treatment decisions. ##

Q176. Answer: A

Explanation: When diet alone fails to control glucose levels, medication is required. This helps maintain normal glucose levels and prevent complications. Delaying treatment increases risk for both mother and fetus. Continuous monitoring is essential. Proper management improves outcomes. ##

Q177. Answer: A

Explanation: Excessive amniotic fluid and large fetal size are characteristic of gestational diabetes. Elevated glucose affects fetal growth and fluid balance. These findings indicate metabolic imbalance. Early management reduces risks. Other conditions do not typically present with both findings. ##

Q178. Answer: A

Explanation: Macrosomia is a key fetal complication of maternal diabetes. Increased glucose availability promotes fetal growth. This can lead to delivery complications. Monitoring and control of glucose reduce this risk. Other options are less commonly associated. ##

Q179. Answer: A

Explanation: Neonatal hypoglycemia occurs due to persistent high insulin levels after birth. Once maternal glucose supply stops, insulin continues to lower blood glucose. This leads to hypoglycemia. Early feeding and monitoring are essential. Other options are not typical outcomes. ##

Q180. Answer: A

Explanation: Poorly controlled diabetes leads to polyhydramnios and macrosomia. Increased fetal urination causes excess amniotic fluid. Large fetal size contributes to maternal discomfort and breathing difficulty. These findings indicate metabolic imbalance. Proper management is required to reduce complications. ##

Q181. Answer: A

Explanation: Fetal hyperinsulinemia occurs due to exposure to high maternal glucose levels in gestational diabetes. The fetus responds by producing excess insulin. This contributes to increased growth and metabolic effects. Other conditions do not lead to this mechanism. Proper maternal glucose control helps prevent this outcome. ##

Q182. Answer: A

Explanation: The confirmatory glucose tolerance test for gestational diabetes is conducted over 3 hours. It involves multiple blood glucose measurements after glucose ingestion. This helps establish a definitive diagnosis. Shorter tests are used for screening only. Accurate diagnosis ensures proper treatment. ##

Q183. Answer: A

Explanation: High maternal glucose leads to increased fetal insulin secretion. Insulin acts as a growth hormone, promoting fat and tissue deposition. This results in macrosomia. Other mechanisms do not explain this growth pattern. Controlling maternal glucose helps reduce this effect. ##

Q184. Answer: A

Explanation: In gestational diabetes, elevated glucose leads to fetal osmotic diuresis. This increases urine production and amniotic fluid volume. The result is polyhydramnios. Other conditions do not typically cause this mechanism. Monitoring fluid levels is important for management. ##

Q185. Answer: C

Explanation: When dietary measures fail to control glucose, pharmacologic therapy is required. This ensures maintenance of normal glucose levels. Delaying treatment increases risks for complications. Continued monitoring is essential. Proper management improves maternal and fetal outcomes. ##

Q186. Answer: B

Explanation: Large fetal size, or macrosomia, increases risk during delivery. It can lead to complications such as difficult labor and injury. Monitoring fetal growth helps guide delivery planning. Small size is associated with different risks. Early intervention reduces complications. ##

Q187. Answer: B

Explanation: Increased fetal urination occurs due to elevated glucose levels in gestational diabetes. This leads to excess amniotic fluid, known as polyhydramnios. The mechanism involves osmotic diuresis. Other options do not explain fluid increase. Managing glucose helps control this condition. ##

Q188. Answer: B

Explanation: Neonatal hypoglycemia occurs due to persistent fetal hyperinsulinemia after birth. The sudden removal of maternal glucose supply leads to low blood sugar. Early feeding and monitoring are essential. Other listed conditions are less common. Proper prenatal control reduces risk. ##

Q189. Answer: A

Explanation: Maintaining normal blood glucose levels is the primary goal of treatment. This reduces complications for both mother and fetus. Proper control prevents macrosomia and metabolic issues. Monitoring is essential throughout pregnancy. Other options are not treatment goals. ##

Q190. Answer: A

Explanation: Poor glucose control leads to polyhydramnios and macrosomia. Increased fetal urination contributes to excess fluid. Large fetal size causes abdominal distension and discomfort. These findings reflect metabolic imbalance. Proper management is required to prevent complications. ##

Q191. Answer: B

Explanation: Macrosomia refers to excessive fetal growth commonly seen in diabetic pregnancies. Elevated maternal glucose leads to increased fetal insulin secretion. Insulin promotes fat deposition and growth. This condition increases delivery complications. Other terms describe reduced or abnormal growth patterns. ##

Q192. Answer: A

Explanation: The glucose challenge test is used as the initial screening tool for gestational diabetes. It involves a fixed glucose load and a single blood measurement. Abnormal results require further testing. It is simple and widely used. Other tests are used for confirmation or different purposes. ##

Q193. Answer: D

Explanation: Insulin acts as a growth-promoting hormone in the fetus. Elevated glucose levels stimulate increased insulin production. This leads to fat accumulation and macrosomia. Other hormones do not play this primary role. Managing maternal glucose helps reduce this effect. ##

Q194. Answer: A

Explanation: Increased fetal urination due to hyperglycemia leads to polyhydramnios. This is caused by osmotic diuresis. The fetus excretes excess glucose through urine. This increases amniotic fluid volume. Other options do not explain fluid increase in this context. ##

Q195. Answer: D

Explanation: When diet alone is insufficient, pharmacologic therapy is required to control glucose levels. This helps prevent complications such as macrosomia. Continuous monitoring guides treatment effectiveness. Delaying treatment increases risks. Proper management improves outcomes for both mother and fetus. ##

Q196. Answer: D

Explanation: Increased fetal size raises the risk of complications such as shoulder dystocia. It makes vaginal delivery more difficult. Monitoring fetal growth helps determine delivery planning. Reduced weight presents different risks. Early intervention reduces complications. ##

Q197. Answer: D

Explanation: Elevated glucose leads to increased fetal urination, causing polyhydramnios. This occurs through osmotic diuresis. The fetus excretes excess glucose in urine. Other mechanisms do not explain increased fluid volume. Managing glucose helps reduce this complication. ##

Q198. Answer: A

Explanation: Neonatal hypoglycemia occurs due to persistent high insulin levels after birth. Once maternal glucose supply stops, insulin lowers blood sugar. This requires early feeding and monitoring. Other conditions are less directly related. Proper prenatal management reduces this risk. ##

Q199. Answer: A

Explanation: Maintaining normal glucose levels is the primary goal of treatment. This reduces risks such as macrosomia and metabolic complications. Monitoring ensures effective control. Other options are not treatment goals. Proper management improves pregnancy outcomes. ##

Q200. Answer: D

Explanation: Poor glucose control leads to macrosomia and polyhydramnios. Increased fetal urination contributes to excess fluid. Large fetal size causes abdominal distension and breathing discomfort. These findings reflect metabolic imbalance. Early intervention is necessary to reduce complications. ##

Question (201-300)

Question (201-300)

Q201. Fetal macrosomia is primarily caused by which metabolic effect in diabetic pregnancy?
(A) Reduced fetal metabolism
(B) Increased insulin activity
(C) Impaired circulation
(D) Decreased glucose transfer

Q202. The glucose tolerance test used for diagnosis of gestational diabetes includes how many hours of monitoring?
(A) Three hour duration
(B) One hour duration
(C) Two hour duration
(D) Four hour duration

Q203. Increased amniotic fluid in diabetic pregnancy is mainly due to which fetal mechanism?
(A) Impaired nutrient transfer
(B) Decreased circulation flow
(C) Increased urinary output
(D) Reduced swallowing activity

Q204. Newborns of diabetic mothers commonly develop which metabolic issue shortly after birth?
(A) Early hypoglycemia
(B) Elevated temperature
(C) Increased blood pressure
(D) Persistent hyperglycemia

Q205. A pregnant woman with gestational diabetes shows persistent hyperglycemia despite dietary measures. What is the next step in care?
(A) Stop monitoring glucose
(B) Delay further action
(C) Continue diet alone
(D) Begin pharmacologic therapy

Q206. A pregnant patient is evaluated before delivery and found to have a significantly large fetus. What complication should be anticipated during labor?
(A) Weak uterine tone
(B) Reduced contractions
(C) Shoulder dystocia
(D) Delayed dilation

Q207. A pregnant woman with diabetes is noted to have increased amniotic fluid and fetal growth on ultrasound. What combined condition does this suggest?
(A) Growth restriction with oligohydramnios
(B) Normal variation pattern
(C) Reduced fetal activity
(D) Macrosomia with polyhydramnios

Q208. A pregnant patient is counseled regarding long-term effects after gestational diabetes. Which risk should be emphasized?
(A) Persistent infection risk
(B) Chronic anemia development
(C) Development of type 2 diabetes
(D) Neurological disorder risk

Q209. A pregnant woman is diagnosed with gestational diabetes and begins treatment. What is the primary goal of therapy?
(A) Maintain normal glucose levels
(B) Enhance fetal growth
(C) Reduce uterine activity
(D) Delay onset of labor
Q210. A pregnant woman with uncontrolled diabetes presents with abdominal distension, breathing difficulty, and ultrasound findings of excessive fluid and large fetus. What is the most likely explanation for her symptoms?
(A) Polyhydramnios with macrosomia
(B) Growth restriction process
(C) Reduced fetal activity pattern
(D) Normal physiological changes
Q211. Which fetal effect is directly caused by elevated maternal glucose levels?
(A) Decreased fat storage
(B) Increased insulin production
(C) Reduced oxygen demand
(D) Impaired circulation
Q212. The screening test for gestational diabetes is typically performed using which method?
(A) Glucose challenge test
(B) Urine glucose test
(C) Random glucose test
(D) Fasting glucose test
Q213. Fetal macrosomia increases the likelihood of which intrapartum complication?
(A) Delayed cervical change
(B) Shoulder dystocia
(C) Decreased uterine tone
(D) Reduced contractions
Q214. Increased amniotic fluid in diabetic pregnancy is primarily due to which process?
(A) Reduced fetal swallowing
(B) Decreased placental flow
(C) Impaired maternal hydration
(D) Increased fetal urination
Q215. A pregnant patient has persistent elevated glucose levels despite diet control. What is the most appropriate next intervention?
(A) Continue diet only
(B) Start medication therapy
(C) Stop glucose checks
(D) Delay treatment plan
Q216. A pregnant woman with diabetes undergoes ultrasound showing excessive fluid and large fetal size. What condition does this indicate?
(A) Macrosomia with polyhydramnios
(B) Reduced fetal movement
(C) Growth restriction pattern
(D) Normal pregnancy variation
Q217. A pregnant patient is counseled after diagnosis of gestational diabetes. Which long-term maternal risk should be addressed?
(A) Type 2 diabetes

(B) Neurological disease
(C) Persistent anemia
(D) Chronic infection

Q218. A pregnant woman presents with a large fetus on examination. What metabolic factor contributes most to this finding?

(A) Increased fetal insulin
(B) Reduced maternal glucose
(C) Decreased placental flow
(D) Impaired fetal metabolism

Q219. A pregnant patient with diabetes is monitored closely during pregnancy. What is the primary goal of this monitoring?

(A) Delay labor onset
(B) Maintain glucose control
(C) Increase fetal size
(D) Reduce uterine activity

Q220. A pregnant woman with uncontrolled diabetes presents with abdominal distension, breathing discomfort, and ultrasound findings of excess fluid and a large fetus. What is the most likely explanation for her symptoms?

(A) Polyhydramnios with macrosomia
(B) Growth restriction pattern
(C) Normal pregnancy changes
(D) Reduced fetal activity

Q221. Fetal hyperinsulinemia in diabetic pregnancy leads primarily to which outcome?

(A) Increased fat deposition
(B) Reduced oxygen demand
(C) Impaired circulation
(D) Decreased growth rate

Q222. The purpose of the glucose challenge test in pregnancy is to do what?

(A) Evaluate placental size
(B) Screen for glucose intolerance
(C) Measure fetal growth
(D) Confirm diabetes diagnosis

Q223. Increased fetal urination in diabetic pregnancy results in which complication?

(A) Oligohydramnios
(B) Polyhydramnios
(C) Growth restriction
(D) Reduced circulation

Q224. Neonatal hypoglycemia after birth in infants of diabetic mothers is caused by what mechanism?

(A) Reduced insulin levels
(B) Persistent high insulin
(C) Decreased glucose use
(D) Increased oxygen demand

Q225. A pregnant woman with gestational diabetes continues to have elevated glucose levels despite diet changes. What is the next step?

(A) Continue observation only
(B) Delay further intervention
(C) Stop glucose monitoring
(D) Initiate pharmacologic treatment

Q226. A pregnant patient with diabetes is evaluated near term and found to have a large fetus. What delivery risk is most significant?
(A) Reduced contractions
(B) Delayed dilation
(C) Shoulder dystocia
(D) Preterm rupture
Q227. A pregnant woman undergoes ultrasound showing increased amniotic fluid and fetal size. What is the most likely underlying condition?
(A) Mild infection
(B) Nutritional deficiency
(C) Gestational diabetes
(D) Chronic hypertension
Q228. A pregnant patient is educated about long-term health after gestational diabetes. Which outcome should be emphasized?
(A) Type 2 diabetes
(B) Recurrent infection
(C) Neurological disease
(D) Chronic anemia
Q229. A pregnant woman with gestational diabetes is undergoing treatment. What is the primary objective of care?
(A) Reduce uterine activity
(B) Increase fetal weight
(C) Delay labor onset
(D) Maintain normal glucose
Q230. A pregnant woman with uncontrolled diabetes presents with abdominal distension, breathing discomfort, and ultrasound findings of excess fluid and large fetus. What is the most likely explanation for her condition?
(A) Normal physiological change
(B) Reduced fetal activity
(C) Growth restriction pattern
(D) Polyhydramnios with macrosomia
Q231. Fetal overgrowth in diabetic pregnancy is mainly due to which hormone effect?
(A) Cortisol reduction effect
(B) Insulin growth effect
(C) Glucagon suppression effect
(D) Thyroid imbalance effect
Q232. The glucose challenge test in pregnancy is used for what purpose?
(A) Measure placental size
(B) Assess fetal growth
(C) Confirm diagnosis
(D) Screen for diabetes
Q233. Excess amniotic fluid in diabetic pregnancy is caused primarily by what fetal activity?
(A) Increased urination
(B) Reduced swallowing
(C) Decreased breathing
(D) Impaired movement
Q234. Infants of diabetic mothers commonly develop which condition after birth?
(A) Hypertension

(B) Hyperglycemia
(C) Hypoglycemia
(D) Hyperthermia

Q235. A pregnant patient with gestational diabetes shows persistent hyperglycemia despite dietary control. What is the next best intervention?
(A) Delay intervention
(B) Initiate medication therapy
(C) Continue diet only
(D) Stop monitoring

Q236. A pregnant woman near term is found to have a large fetus on ultrasound. What labor complication should be anticipated?
(A) Shoulder dystocia
(B) Delayed dilation
(C) Weak uterine tone
(D) Reduced contractions

Q237. A pregnant patient has increased amniotic fluid and fetal size on imaging. What underlying condition is most likely present?
(A) Nutritional deficiency
(B) Mild infection
(C) Gestational diabetes
(D) Chronic anemia

Q238. A pregnant woman is counseled about long-term risks after gestational diabetes. Which condition should be highlighted?
(A) Chronic infection
(B) Neurological disorder
(C) Persistent anemia
(D) Type 2 diabetes

Q239. A pregnant patient is undergoing treatment for gestational diabetes. What is the primary goal of management?
(A) Delay labor onset
(B) Reduce uterine activity
(C) Maintain glucose control
(D) Increase fetal size

Q240. A pregnant woman with uncontrolled diabetes presents with abdominal distension, shortness of breath, and ultrasound findings of excess fluid and large fetus. What is the most likely explanation for her condition?
(A) Normal pregnancy adaptation
(B) Polyhydramnios with macrosomia
(C) Reduced fetal activity
(D) Growth restriction process

Q241. Fetal macrosomia in diabetic pregnancy is driven mainly by which process?
(A) Increased insulin secretion
(B) Decreased nutrient supply
(C) Reduced glucose transfer
(D) Impaired circulation

Q242. The confirmatory test for gestational diabetes evaluates glucose levels over what period?
(A) Four hour duration
(B) One hour duration

(C) Three hour duration
(D) Two hour duration
Q243. Increased fetal urine production in diabetic pregnancy leads to which condition?
(A) Polyhydramnios
(B) Reduced circulation
(C) Growth restriction
(D) Oligohydramnios
Q244. Neonatal hypoglycemia in infants of diabetic mothers is caused by what factor?
(A) Increased metabolism
(B) Reduced glucose use
(C) High insulin levels
(D) Low insulin levels
Q245. A pregnant woman with gestational diabetes has uncontrolled glucose despite diet therapy. What is the next step?
(A) Continue diet alone
(B) Stop monitoring
(C) Start medication therapy
(D) Delay intervention
Q246. A pregnant patient is found to have a large fetus near term. What complication should the healthcare provider anticipate?
(A) Delayed dilation
(B) Weak uterine tone
(C) Shoulder dystocia
(D) Reduced contractions
Q247. A pregnant woman has ultrasound findings of excessive amniotic fluid and large fetal size. What condition is most likely responsible?
(A) Nutritional deficiency
(B) Mild anemia
(C) Chronic infection
(D) Gestational diabetes
Q248. A pregnant patient is educated about future health risks after gestational diabetes. Which risk is most significant?
(A) Type 2 diabetes
(B) Neurological disease
(C) Recurrent infection
(D) Chronic anemia
Q249. A pregnant woman undergoing treatment for gestational diabetes has a primary goal of maintaining what?
(A) Increased fetal growth
(B) Delayed labor onset
(C) Reduced uterine activity
(D) Normal glucose levels
Q250. A pregnant woman with poorly controlled diabetes presents with abdominal distension, breathing discomfort, and ultrasound findings of excessive fluid and a large fetus. What condition best explains these findings?
(A) Reduced fetal activity
(B) Polyhydramnios with macrosomia
(C) Normal physiological change

(D) Growth restriction pattern
Q251. Excess fetal growth due to maternal diabetes is mainly linked to which fetal hormone action?
(A) Thyroid imbalance effect
(B) Insulin stimulation effect
(C) Glucagon suppression effect
(D) Cortisol reduction effect
Q252. The glucose tolerance test used for diagnosis evaluates blood glucose over which time frame?
(A) Four hour interval
(B) Three hour interval
(C) Two hour interval
(D) One hour interval
Q253. Increased amniotic fluid volume in diabetic pregnancy results from which fetal process?
(A) Decreased circulation flow
(B) Increased urinary output
(C) Reduced swallowing action
(D) Impaired oxygen exchange
Q254. Neonatal hypoglycemia following delivery is primarily due to what condition?
(A) High insulin levels
(B) Low insulin levels
(C) Reduced glucose intake
(D) Increased metabolism
Q255. A pregnant woman with gestational diabetes continues to have elevated glucose despite diet therapy. What is the most appropriate next step?
(A) Continue dietary plan only
(B) Stop glucose monitoring
(C) Initiate pharmacologic therapy
(D) Delay further intervention
Q256. A pregnant patient is assessed near term and found to have a large fetus. What complication is most likely during labor?
(A) Delayed cervical change
(B) Reduced contraction pattern
(C) Weak uterine tone pattern
(D) Shoulder dystocia event
Q257. A pregnant woman presents with ultrasound findings of increased amniotic fluid and large fetal size. What is the most likely underlying condition?
(A) Mild infection process
(B) Gestational diabetes condition
(C) Chronic hypertension disorder
(D) Nutritional deficiency state
Q258. A pregnant patient is counseled regarding long-term health after gestational diabetes. Which risk is most significant?
(A) Type 2 diabetes risk
(B) Chronic anemia development
(C) Recurrent infection risk
(D) Neurological disorder risk
Q259. A pregnant woman undergoing treatment for gestational diabetes has a primary goal of maintaining what outcome?
(A) Normal maternal glucose level

(B) Reduced uterine activity
(C) Increased fetal growth rate
(D) Delayed onset of labor

Q260. A pregnant woman with poorly controlled diabetes presents with abdominal distension, breathing discomfort, and ultrasound findings of excessive fluid and a large fetus. What is the most likely explanation for these findings?

(A) Growth restriction pattern
(B) Normal physiological adaptation
(C) Polyhydramnios with macrosomia
(D) Reduced fetal activity pattern

Q261. Excess fetal growth in diabetic pregnancy is primarily caused by which fetal response?

(A) Impaired circulation flow
(B) Increased insulin secretion
(C) Decreased oxygen demand
(D) Reduced glucose transfer

Q262. The diagnostic glucose tolerance test for gestational diabetes typically spans what duration?

(A) One hour duration
(B) Two hour duration
(C) Four hour duration
(D) Three hour duration

Q263. A postpartum patient preparing for discharge reports concerns about breastfeeding effectiveness, recognizing newborn complications, safe sleep practices, and managing care independently due to limited support, while also showing anxiety and repeated misunderstanding despite multiple teaching sessions; the nurse reassesses readiness and identifies persistent knowledge deficits. What is the most appropriate nursing action in this situation?

(A) Delay discharge without explanation
(B) Refer without additional education
(C) Provide structured repeated teaching and support
(D) Avoid addressing concerns

Q264. Neonatal hypoglycemia after birth is primarily caused by which factor in infants of diabetic mothers?

(A) Increased oxygen use
(B) High insulin level
(C) Low insulin level
(D) Reduced metabolism rate

Q265. A pregnant woman with gestational diabetes has persistent hyperglycemia despite dietary changes. What is the next appropriate management step?

(A) Stop glucose monitoring
(B) Delay further care
(C) Initiate medication therapy
(D) Continue diet alone

Q266. A pregnant patient near term is found to have a large fetus on examination. What complication should be anticipated during labor?

(A) Reduced contraction strength
(B) Delayed cervical dilation
(C) Shoulder dystocia event
(D) Weak uterine tone pattern

Q267. A pregnant woman has ultrasound findings of excessive amniotic fluid and increased fetal size. What is the most likely underlying condition?
(A) Chronic anemia disorder
(B) Nutritional deficiency state
(C) Gestational diabetes condition
(D) Mild infection process
Q268. A pregnant patient is counseled about long-term outcomes after gestational diabetes. Which condition is most important to monitor?
(A) Recurrent infection risk
(B) Neurological disorder risk
(C) Chronic anemia risk
(D) Type 2 diabetes risk
Q269. A pregnant woman receiving treatment for gestational diabetes aims to achieve what primary outcome?
(A) Delayed onset of labor
(B) Reduced uterine activity
(C) Normal maternal glucose level
(D) Increased fetal growth rate
Q270. A pregnant woman with uncontrolled diabetes presents with abdominal distension, breathing difficulty, and ultrasound findings of excess amniotic fluid and a large fetus. What is the most likely explanation for her symptoms?
(A) Normal pregnancy adaptation
(B) Reduced fetal activity pattern
(C) Polyhydramnios with macrosomia
(D) Growth restriction condition
Q271. Fetal overgrowth in diabetic pregnancy is primarily linked to which mechanism?
(A) Impaired placental flow
(B) Decreased nutrient supply
(C) Reduced glucose transfer
(D) Increased insulin secretion
Q272. The glucose tolerance test used for diagnosis measures glucose over what period?
(A) Two hour duration
(B) Three hour duration
(C) Four hour duration
(D) One hour duration
Q273. Polyhydramnios in diabetic pregnancy is mainly caused by which fetal process?
(A) Decreased circulation flow
(B) Impaired oxygen exchange
(C) Reduced swallowing action
(D) Increased urine production
Q274. Neonatal hypoglycemia occurs in infants of diabetic mothers due to which condition?
(A) Low insulin level
(B) Reduced glucose intake
(C) High insulin level
(D) Increased metabolism rate
Q275. A pregnant woman with gestational diabetes has elevated glucose despite diet therapy. What is the next step?
(A) Stop glucose checks

(B) Delay further action
(C) Initiate medication therapy
(D) Continue diet alone

Q276. A pregnant patient is found to have a large fetus near term. What complication should be anticipated during delivery?
(A) Weak uterine tone pattern
(B) Reduced contraction strength
(C) Delayed cervical dilation
(D) Shoulder dystocia event

Q277. A pregnant woman presents with increased amniotic fluid and fetal size on ultrasound. What underlying condition is most likely?
(A) Mild infection process
(B) Gestational diabetes condition
(C) Chronic anemia disorder
(D) Nutritional deficiency state

Q278. A pregnant patient is counseled on long-term risks after gestational diabetes. Which risk is most significant?
(A) Type 2 diabetes risk
(B) Recurrent infection risk
(C) Chronic anemia development
(D) Neurological disorder risk

Q279. A pregnant woman undergoing treatment for gestational diabetes aims to achieve which primary goal?
(A) Normal glucose control
(B) Increased fetal growth rate
(C) Delayed onset of labor
(D) Reduced uterine activity

Q280. A pregnant woman with uncontrolled diabetes presents with abdominal distension, breathing difficulty, and ultrasound findings of excessive fluid and a large fetus. What is the most likely explanation for her symptoms?
(A) Growth restriction condition
(B) Normal physiological adaptation
(C) Reduced fetal activity pattern
(D) Polyhydramnios with macrosomia

Q281. Fetal macrosomia in diabetic pregnancy results primarily from which fetal response?
(A) Decreased metabolism rate
(B) Reduced glucose transfer
(C) Increased insulin production
(D) Impaired placental flow

Q282. The diagnostic glucose tolerance test in pregnancy is conducted over what time period?
(A) Two hour duration
(B) One hour duration
(C) Three hour duration
(D) Four hour duration

Q283. Polyhydramnios in diabetic pregnancy is primarily due to which fetal mechanism?
(A) Reduced swallowing action
(B) Increased urine production
(C) Decreased oxygen delivery

(D) Impaired circulation flow

Q284. Neonatal hypoglycemia after birth is mainly caused by which factor in infants of diabetic mothers?

(A) Reduced glucose intake
(B) Low insulin level
(C) High insulin level
(D) Increased metabolism rate

Q285. A pregnant woman with gestational diabetes has persistent hyperglycemia despite dietary management. What is the next appropriate step?

(A) Stop glucose monitoring
(B) Continue diet only
(C) Initiate medication therapy
(D) Delay intervention

Q286. A pregnant patient near term is found to have a large fetus. What complication is most likely during labor?

(A) Shoulder dystocia event
(B) Weak uterine tone pattern
(C) Reduced contraction strength
(D) Delayed cervical dilation

Q287. A pregnant woman presents with increased amniotic fluid and fetal size on ultrasound. What underlying condition is most likely responsible?

(A) Mild infection process
(B) Chronic anemia disorder
(C) Nutritional deficiency state
(D) Gestational diabetes condition

Q288. A pregnant patient is counseled about long-term risks after gestational diabetes. Which condition should be emphasized?

(A) Type 2 diabetes risk
(B) Recurrent infection risk
(C) Neurological disorder risk
(D) Chronic anemia development

Q289. A newborn demonstrates decreased tone, weak cry, and irregular respirations immediately after birth but improves quickly after stimulation, warming, and airway support within minutes; what does this indicate about neonatal transition?

(A) Severe respiratory failure
(B) Circulatory collapse
(C) Mild transitional difficulty
(D) Neurological impairment

Q290. A pregnant woman with uncontrolled diabetes presents with abdominal distension, breathing discomfort, and ultrasound findings of excessive fluid and a large fetus. What is the most likely explanation for her condition?

(A) Normal pregnancy adaptation
(B) Reduced fetal activity pattern
(C) Growth restriction condition
(D) Polyhydramnios with macrosomia

Q291. Fetal overgrowth in diabetic pregnancy is mainly due to which effect?

(A) Decreased oxygen demand
(B) Impaired placental flow

(C) Reduced glucose supply
(D) Increased insulin activity
Q292. The glucose tolerance test confirms gestational diabetes by measuring glucose over what duration?
(A) Two hour period
(B) Four hour period
(C) One hour period
(D) Three hour period
Q293. Polyhydramnios in diabetic pregnancy results primarily from which fetal process?
(A) Reduced swallowing reflex
(B) Decreased circulation flow
(C) Impaired oxygen exchange
(D) Increased urine output
Q294. Neonatal hypoglycemia in infants of diabetic mothers is caused by what condition?
(A) Reduced glucose intake
(B) High insulin level
(C) Low insulin level
(D) Increased metabolism rate
Q295. A pregnant woman with gestational diabetes continues to have elevated glucose levels despite diet therapy. What is the next step in management?
(A) Stop glucose monitoring
(B) Delay further action
(C) Continue diet only
(D) Initiate medication therapy
Q296. A nurse observes a colleague failing to verify patient identity before administering medication to a newborn, increasing risk of error; what is the most appropriate professional action?
(A) Ignore the behavior
(B) Report according to safety protocol
(C) Document similar practice
(D) Confront without escalation
Q297. A postpartum patient exclusively pumping breast milk reports decreasing supply after inconsistent pumping intervals and skipped sessions due to fatigue and workload; what is the most appropriate nursing recommendation?
(A) Maintain regular frequent pumping
(B) Avoid nighttime pumping
(C) Reduce pumping sessions further
(D) Stop pumping temporarily
Q298. A pregnant patient is counseled about long-term health after gestational diabetes. Which condition should be emphasized?
(A) Neurological disorder risk
(B) Type 2 diabetes risk
(C) Chronic anemia development
(D) Recurrent infection risk
Q299. A newborn develops rapid breathing, nasal flaring, and intercostal retractions with decreasing oxygen saturation despite initial stabilization; what condition is most likely present?
(A) Respiratory distress condition
(B) Thermoregulation imbalance
(C) Normal transition process

(D) Feeding difficulty issue

Q300. A pregnant woman with uncontrolled diabetes presents with abdominal distension, breathing difficulty, and ultrasound findings of excessive amniotic fluid and a large fetus. What is the most likely explanation for her symptoms?

(A) Growth restriction condition
(B) Polyhydramnios with macrosomia
(C) Reduced fetal activity pattern
(D) Normal pregnancy adaptation

Answer Key and Explanation (201-300)

Q201. Answer: B

Explanation: In diabetic pregnancy, elevated maternal glucose crosses the placenta and stimulates fetal insulin production. Insulin acts as a growth hormone, leading to increased fat deposition and macrosomia. This metabolic effect is central to excessive fetal growth. Other mechanisms do not explain this pattern. Proper glucose control reduces this risk. ##

Q202. Answer: A

Explanation: The diagnostic glucose tolerance test typically measures blood glucose levels over a 3-hour period. This allows evaluation of how the body processes glucose over time. Multiple readings improve diagnostic accuracy. Shorter tests are used for screening purposes. This test confirms gestational diabetes diagnosis. ##

Q203. Answer: C

Explanation: Elevated fetal glucose levels lead to osmotic diuresis, increasing urinary output. This results in excess amniotic fluid, known as polyhydramnios. The mechanism is directly linked to maternal hyperglycemia. Other options do not explain fluid accumulation in this condition. Monitoring is essential for management. ##

Q204. Answer: A

Explanation: Neonatal hypoglycemia occurs due to persistent fetal hyperinsulinemia after birth. Once maternal glucose supply is removed, insulin continues to lower blood glucose levels. This results in hypoglycemia. Early feeding and monitoring are essential. Other metabolic issues are less directly associated. ##

Q205. Answer: D

Explanation: When diet alone fails to control glucose, pharmacologic therapy is required. This helps maintain normal glucose levels and reduce complications. Continuous monitoring guides therapy adjustments. Delaying treatment increases maternal and fetal risks. Early intervention improves overall outcomes. ##

Q206. Answer: C

Explanation: A large fetus increases the risk of shoulder dystocia during delivery. This occurs when the fetal shoulders fail to pass easily through the birth canal. It can lead to complications for both mother and baby. Monitoring fetal size helps in planning delivery. Early recognition reduces risk. ##

Q207. Answer: D

Explanation: Diabetes can cause both macrosomia and polyhydramnios simultaneously. Increased glucose leads to fetal hyperinsulinemia and growth, while osmotic diuresis increases fluid. These findings indicate metabolic imbalance. Close monitoring is required. Proper management reduces complications. ##

Q208. Answer: C

Explanation: Women with gestational diabetes have a significantly increased risk of developing type 2 diabetes later in life. This risk persists beyond pregnancy. Lifestyle changes and follow-up screening are important. Early intervention can reduce progression. Other conditions are not primary long-term risks. ##

Q209. Answer: A

Explanation: The primary goal is to maintain normal maternal glucose levels. This prevents complications such as macrosomia and neonatal hypoglycemia. Monitoring ensures effective control. Treatment may include diet, exercise, and medication. Achieving glycemic control improves maternal and fetal outcomes. ##

Q210. Answer: A

Explanation: Poorly controlled diabetes leads to polyhydramnios and macrosomia. Increased fetal urination causes fluid accumulation, while insulin-driven growth enlarges the fetus. These factors contribute to maternal discomfort and breathing difficulty. This reflects metabolic imbalance. Early management is essential to reduce complications. ##

Q211. Answer: B

Explanation: Elevated maternal glucose crosses the placenta and stimulates fetal insulin production. This leads to hyperinsulinemia, which promotes growth and fat deposition. It is a key mechanism behind macrosomia. Other options do not describe this metabolic effect. Proper glucose control reduces fetal complications. ##

Q212. Answer: A

Explanation: The glucose challenge test is the standard screening tool for gestational diabetes. It involves administering a glucose load and measuring blood sugar after one hour. It does not require fasting. Abnormal results lead to confirmatory testing. Other tests are not used for initial screening. ##

Q213. Answer: B

Explanation: Macrosomia leads to increased risk of shoulder dystocia during labor. The large fetal size makes delivery through the birth canal more difficult. This can result in injury if not managed appropriately. Early identification allows planning of delivery. Other options are not directly linked. ##

Q214. Answer: D

Explanation: Elevated fetal glucose leads to osmotic diuresis, causing increased urination. This results in polyhydramnios. The mechanism is directly related to maternal hyperglycemia. Other processes do not explain the fluid increase. Monitoring fluid levels is essential for management. ##

Q215. Answer: B

Explanation: When dietary measures fail to control glucose levels, pharmacologic therapy is required. This helps maintain euglycemia and prevent complications. Continued monitoring ensures treatment effectiveness. Delaying intervention increases risk for both mother and fetus. Proper management improves outcomes. ##

Q216. Answer: A

Explanation: The combination of excessive amniotic fluid and large fetal size is characteristic of diabetic pregnancy. Increased fetal urination leads to polyhydramnios, while hyperinsulinemia causes macrosomia. These findings indicate metabolic imbalance. Close monitoring is necessary. Early management reduces complications. ##

Q217. Answer: A

Explanation: Gestational diabetes significantly increases the risk of developing type 2 diabetes later in life. This risk persists long after pregnancy. Follow-up screening and lifestyle changes are important. Early intervention can reduce progression. Other options are not primary long-term risks. ##

Q218. Answer: A

Explanation: Increased fetal insulin production drives excessive growth in diabetic pregnancies. Insulin promotes fat deposition and tissue growth. This results in macrosomia. Other factors do not explain this pattern. Managing maternal glucose reduces this effect. ##

Q219. Answer: B

Explanation: The primary goal is to maintain normal blood glucose levels. This reduces risks such as macrosomia and neonatal hypoglycemia. Monitoring allows timely adjustments in therapy. Proper control improves maternal and fetal outcomes. Other options are not primary goals. ##

Q220. Answer: A

Explanation: Poorly controlled diabetes leads to increased fetal urination and growth. This results in polyhydramnios and macrosomia. These changes cause abdominal distension and respiratory discomfort. The condition reflects metabolic imbalance. Early intervention is necessary to prevent complications. ##

Q221. Answer: A
Explanation: Fetal hyperinsulinemia promotes fat deposition and tissue growth, leading to macrosomia. Elevated maternal glucose stimulates insulin production in the fetus. Insulin acts as a growth hormone in this context. Other options do not reflect the metabolic effect. Proper glucose control helps prevent this outcome. ##
Q222. Answer: B
Explanation: The glucose challenge test is used as a screening tool for gestational diabetes. It identifies individuals who may have glucose intolerance. Abnormal results require confirmatory testing. It is not used to confirm diagnosis. Early screening helps detect and manage the condition effectively. ##
Q223. Answer: B
Explanation: Increased fetal urination due to elevated glucose levels leads to polyhydramnios. This occurs through osmotic diuresis. The fetus excretes excess glucose via urine. This increases amniotic fluid volume. Other options do not describe this condition. Monitoring is essential for management. ##
Q224. Answer: B
Explanation: Neonatal hypoglycemia occurs because the fetus produces high insulin levels in response to maternal glucose. After birth, glucose supply stops but insulin remains elevated. This lowers blood glucose levels. Early feeding is necessary to correct it. Other options do not explain this mechanism. ##
Q225. Answer: D
Explanation: Persistent hyperglycemia despite diet requires pharmacologic intervention. This ensures proper glucose control and reduces complications. Monitoring helps assess effectiveness. Delaying treatment increases risks. Early management improves maternal and fetal outcomes. ##
Q226. Answer: C
Explanation: A large fetus increases the risk of shoulder dystocia during delivery. This can lead to complications such as birth injury. Monitoring fetal size helps guide delivery planning. Early identification allows appropriate management. Other options are not directly related to macrosomia. ##
Q227. Answer: C
Explanation: Gestational diabetes commonly leads to both polyhydramnios and macrosomia. Elevated glucose levels affect fetal metabolism and fluid balance. These findings indicate metabolic imbalance. Early diagnosis allows proper management. Other conditions do not typically present with both findings. ##
Q228. Answer: A
Explanation: Gestational diabetes increases the risk of developing type 2 diabetes later in life. This risk remains significant after pregnancy. Follow-up care and lifestyle changes are important. Early detection can prevent complications. Other conditions are not primary long-term outcomes. ##
Q229. Answer: D
Explanation: Maintaining normal blood glucose levels is the primary objective. This prevents complications such as macrosomia and neonatal hypoglycemia. Monitoring ensures effective treatment. Proper management improves outcomes. Other options are not treatment goals. ##
Q230. Answer: D
Explanation: Poor glucose control leads to increased fetal urination and growth. This results in polyhydramnios and macrosomia. These changes cause abdominal distension and breathing discomfort. The condition reflects metabolic imbalance. Early intervention is necessary to reduce complications. ##
Q231. Answer: B
Explanation: Insulin acts as a growth-promoting hormone in the fetus. Elevated maternal glucose stimulates fetal insulin secretion. This leads to increased fat storage and tissue growth. The result is macrosomia. Other hormonal effects do not explain this pattern. Proper glucose control helps prevent this outcome. ##
Q232. Answer: D

Explanation: The glucose challenge test is a screening test used to identify women at risk for gestational diabetes. It is not diagnostic. Abnormal results require a glucose tolerance test for confirmation. Early screening allows timely management. Other options are not its purpose. ##

Q233. Answer: A

Explanation: Increased fetal urination occurs due to elevated glucose levels. This results in osmotic diuresis and accumulation of amniotic fluid. The condition is called polyhydramnios. Other activities do not significantly affect fluid volume. Monitoring is essential to manage complications. ##

Q234. Answer: C

Explanation: Neonatal hypoglycemia occurs due to persistent high insulin levels after birth. The sudden removal of maternal glucose supply leads to low blood sugar. Early feeding is required to stabilize levels. Monitoring is essential in the newborn period. Other conditions are less commonly associated. ##

Q235. Answer: B

Explanation: Pharmacologic therapy is required when diet alone fails to control glucose levels. This helps maintain normal glucose levels and reduce complications. Continuous monitoring guides therapy adjustments. Delaying treatment increases risks. Proper management improves outcomes for mother and fetus. ##

Q236. Answer: A

Explanation: A large fetus increases the risk of shoulder dystocia during delivery. This occurs when the shoulders fail to pass easily through the birth canal. It can lead to injury if not managed appropriately. Early recognition helps in planning delivery. Other options are not directly related. ##

Q237. Answer: C

Explanation: Gestational diabetes commonly results in both polyhydramnios and macrosomia. Elevated glucose levels affect fetal metabolism and fluid balance. These findings indicate metabolic imbalance. Early diagnosis allows proper management. Other conditions do not typically cause both findings together. ##

Q238. Answer: D

Explanation: Gestational diabetes increases the risk of developing type 2 diabetes later in life. This risk remains significant after pregnancy. Follow-up screening is important for early detection. Lifestyle changes can reduce progression. Other options are not primary long-term risks. ##

Q239. Answer: C

Explanation: Maintaining normal glucose levels is the main goal of treatment. This reduces risks such as macrosomia and neonatal hypoglycemia. Monitoring ensures effective control. Proper management improves maternal and fetal outcomes. Other options are not treatment goals. ##

Q240. Answer: B

Explanation: Poor glucose control leads to excessive fetal growth and increased amniotic fluid. Increased fetal urination contributes to polyhydramnios. These findings cause abdominal distension and breathing discomfort. The condition reflects metabolic imbalance. Early management is required to prevent complications. ##

Q241. Answer: A

Explanation: Elevated maternal glucose crosses the placenta and stimulates fetal insulin secretion. Insulin acts as a growth hormone, promoting fat deposition and tissue growth. This leads to macrosomia. Other processes do not explain this pattern. Maintaining glucose control reduces this complication. ##

Q242. Answer: C

Explanation: The glucose tolerance test for gestational diabetes measures blood glucose over a 3-hour period. This allows assessment of how the body processes glucose over time. Multiple readings improve diagnostic accuracy. Shorter tests are used for screening only. This test confirms the diagnosis. ##

Q243. Answer: A

Explanation: Increased fetal urination due to high glucose levels causes polyhydramnios. This occurs through osmotic diuresis. Excess glucose is excreted in urine, increasing fluid volume. Other options do not describe this condition. Monitoring is essential to manage risks. ##

Q244. Answer: C

Explanation: High fetal insulin levels persist after birth. When maternal glucose supply stops, insulin lowers blood glucose levels rapidly. This results in hypoglycemia. Early feeding helps stabilize glucose. Monitoring is essential in newborns. Other options do not explain this mechanism. ##

Q245. Answer: C

Explanation: Pharmacologic therapy is required when diet alone does not control glucose levels. This helps maintain normal glucose levels and prevent complications. Continuous monitoring ensures treatment effectiveness. Delaying intervention increases risk. Proper management improves outcomes for both mother and fetus. ##

Q246. Answer: C

Explanation: Macrosomia increases the risk of shoulder dystocia during delivery. This occurs when the fetal shoulders become stuck during birth. It can lead to complications if not managed properly. Early identification helps in planning delivery. Other options are not directly related. ##

Q247. Answer: D

Explanation: Gestational diabetes leads to increased fetal growth and excessive amniotic fluid. Elevated glucose levels affect fetal metabolism and fluid balance. These findings indicate metabolic imbalance. Early diagnosis allows appropriate management. Other conditions do not typically present this way. ##

Q248. Answer: A

Explanation: Women with gestational diabetes have an increased risk of developing type 2 diabetes later in life. This risk persists long after pregnancy. Regular follow-up and lifestyle changes are important. Early detection can prevent complications. Other options are not primary risks. ##

Q249. Answer: D

Explanation: The main goal of treatment is to maintain normal maternal glucose levels. This prevents complications such as macrosomia and neonatal hypoglycemia. Monitoring ensures effective control. Proper management improves maternal and fetal outcomes. Other options are not treatment goals. ##

Q250. Answer: B

Explanation: Poor glucose control leads to increased fetal urination and growth. This results in polyhydramnios and macrosomia. These findings cause abdominal distension and respiratory discomfort. The condition reflects metabolic imbalance. Early management is essential to prevent complications. ##

Q251. Answer: B

Explanation: Elevated maternal glucose leads to increased fetal insulin secretion. Insulin promotes fat storage and tissue growth in the fetus. This results in macrosomia. Other hormonal actions do not produce this growth pattern. Maintaining maternal glucose levels helps reduce this effect. ##

Q252. Answer: B

Explanation: The diagnostic glucose tolerance test measures glucose levels over a 3-hour period. This allows assessment of how the body processes glucose over time. Multiple readings provide accurate diagnosis. Screening tests are shorter in duration. This test confirms gestational diabetes. ##

Q253. Answer: B

Explanation: Elevated glucose causes osmotic diuresis in the fetus, increasing urine production. This leads to polyhydramnios. The excess fluid accumulates in the amniotic sac. Other processes do not significantly increase fluid volume. Monitoring helps detect and manage this condition. ##

Q254. Answer: A

Explanation: Persistent fetal hyperinsulinemia continues after birth. When maternal glucose supply stops, insulin lowers blood glucose levels rapidly. This results in hypoglycemia. Early feeding helps stabilize glucose levels. Monitoring is essential to prevent complications. ##

Q255. Answer: C
Explanation: Pharmacologic therapy is indicated when diet alone does not control glucose levels. This ensures proper glycemic control. Delaying treatment increases risks of complications. Monitoring guides therapy adjustments. Proper management improves outcomes for both mother and fetus. ##
Q256. Answer: D
Explanation: Macrosomia increases the risk of shoulder dystocia during delivery. The fetal shoulders may become impacted during birth. This can lead to complications if not managed appropriately. Early recognition allows planning for safe delivery. Other options are not directly related. ##
Q257. Answer: B
Explanation: Gestational diabetes commonly causes both macrosomia and polyhydramnios. Elevated glucose affects fetal metabolism and fluid balance. These findings indicate metabolic imbalance. Early diagnosis allows appropriate intervention. Other conditions do not typically produce both findings together. ##
Q258. Answer: A
Explanation: Women with gestational diabetes have an increased risk of developing type 2 diabetes later in life. This risk persists after pregnancy. Follow-up screening is essential for early detection. Lifestyle changes can reduce progression. Other conditions are not primary long-term risks. ##
Q259. Answer: A
Explanation: The primary goal is to maintain normal maternal glucose levels. This prevents complications such as macrosomia and neonatal hypoglycemia. Monitoring ensures treatment effectiveness. Proper control improves maternal and fetal outcomes. Other options are not treatment goals. ##
Q260. Answer: C
Explanation: Poor glucose control leads to increased fetal urination and excessive growth. This results in polyhydramnios and macrosomia. These changes cause abdominal distension and breathing discomfort. The condition reflects metabolic imbalance. Early intervention is required to prevent complications. ##
Q261. Answer: B
Explanation: Elevated maternal glucose crosses the placenta and stimulates fetal insulin secretion. Insulin promotes fat deposition and tissue growth. This leads to macrosomia. Other responses do not explain the increased growth pattern. Maintaining maternal glucose levels helps prevent this complication. ##
Q262. Answer: D
Explanation: The glucose tolerance test evaluates blood glucose levels over a 3-hour period. Multiple readings help determine how the body processes glucose. This provides a definitive diagnosis. Shorter tests are used for screening purposes. Accurate diagnosis guides appropriate treatment. ##
Q263. Answer: C
Explanation: Structured repeated teaching reinforces understanding of key concepts. Addressing concerns improves patient confidence. Emotional support reduces anxiety levels. Clear instructions ensure safe newborn care practices. Providing resources helps compensate for limited support. This approach ensures readiness for safe discharge. ##
Q264. Answer: B
Explanation: Fetal hyperinsulinemia persists after birth. When maternal glucose supply stops, insulin continues to lower blood glucose levels. This results in hypoglycemia. Early feeding and monitoring are necessary. Other factors do not explain this condition. Proper prenatal control reduces this risk. ##
Q265. Answer: C
Explanation: When diet alone fails to control glucose levels, pharmacologic therapy is required. This ensures proper glycemic control and reduces complications. Monitoring helps adjust treatment. Delaying intervention increases risks. Early management improves outcomes for both mother and fetus. ##
Q266. Answer: C

Explanation: Macrosomia increases the risk of shoulder dystocia during delivery. The fetal shoulders may become impacted in the birth canal. This can lead to complications if not managed appropriately. Early identification allows for proper planning. Other options are not directly associated. ##

Q267. Answer: C

Explanation: Gestational diabetes commonly results in macrosomia and polyhydramnios. Elevated glucose affects fetal metabolism and fluid balance. These findings indicate metabolic imbalance. Early diagnosis allows for appropriate management. Other conditions do not typically present with both findings together. ##

Q268. Answer: D

Explanation: Women with gestational diabetes have a significantly increased risk of developing type 2 diabetes later in life. This risk persists after pregnancy. Follow-up screening is essential for early detection. Lifestyle modifications can reduce progression. Other options are not primary long-term risks. ##

Q269. Answer: C

Explanation: The main goal of treatment is to maintain normal maternal glucose levels. This reduces risks such as macrosomia and neonatal hypoglycemia. Monitoring ensures effective control. Proper management improves maternal and fetal outcomes. Other options are not treatment goals. ##

Q270. Answer: C

Explanation: Poorly controlled diabetes leads to increased fetal urination and excessive growth. This results in polyhydramnios and macrosomia. These changes cause abdominal distension and breathing difficulty. The condition reflects metabolic imbalance. Early intervention is necessary to prevent complications. ##

Q271. Answer: D

Explanation: Elevated maternal glucose crosses the placenta and stimulates fetal insulin production. Insulin acts as a growth hormone, promoting fat deposition and tissue growth. This leads to macrosomia. Other mechanisms do not explain this growth pattern. Maintaining glucose control reduces this complication. ##

Q272. Answer: B

Explanation: The diagnostic glucose tolerance test measures blood glucose levels over a 3-hour period. This allows evaluation of glucose metabolism over time. Multiple readings increase diagnostic accuracy. Screening tests are shorter. This test confirms gestational diabetes diagnosis. ##

Q273. Answer: D

Explanation: Elevated glucose levels cause osmotic diuresis in the fetus, increasing urine production. This results in polyhydramnios. Excess fluid accumulates in the amniotic sac. Other processes do not significantly affect fluid volume. Monitoring helps detect complications early. ##

Q274. Answer: C

Explanation: Fetal hyperinsulinemia persists after birth. Once maternal glucose supply stops, insulin lowers blood glucose levels. This results in hypoglycemia. Early feeding is required to stabilize levels. Monitoring is essential in newborn care. Other factors do not explain this condition. ##

Q275. Answer: C

Explanation: When diet fails to control glucose levels, pharmacologic therapy is required. This ensures proper glycemic control and reduces complications. Monitoring helps guide treatment adjustments. Delaying intervention increases risks. Early management improves outcomes for mother and fetus. ##

Q276. Answer: D

Explanation: Macrosomia increases the risk of shoulder dystocia. The fetal shoulders may become impacted during delivery. This can lead to complications if not managed appropriately. Early recognition allows proper delivery planning. Other options are not directly related. ##

Q277. Answer: B

Explanation: Gestational diabetes leads to both macrosomia and polyhydramnios. Elevated glucose affects fetal metabolism and fluid balance. These findings indicate metabolic imbalance. Early diagnosis allows appropriate intervention. Other conditions do not typically cause both findings together. ##

Q278. Answer: A

Explanation: Gestational diabetes increases the risk of developing type 2 diabetes later in life. This risk persists beyond pregnancy. Follow-up screening is essential for early detection. Lifestyle modifications can reduce progression. Other options are not primary risks. ##

Q279. Answer: A

Explanation: The primary goal is to maintain normal maternal glucose levels. This prevents complications such as macrosomia and neonatal hypoglycemia. Monitoring ensures effective control. Proper management improves maternal and fetal outcomes. Other options are not treatment goals. ##

Q280. Answer: D

Explanation: Poor glucose control leads to increased fetal urination and excessive growth. This results in polyhydramnios and macrosomia. These changes cause abdominal distension and breathing difficulty. The condition reflects metabolic imbalance. Early intervention is necessary to prevent complications. ##

Q281. Answer: C

Explanation: Elevated maternal glucose stimulates fetal insulin production. Insulin promotes fat deposition and tissue growth in the fetus. This leads to macrosomia. Other responses do not account for excessive growth. Maintaining glucose control helps reduce this complication. ##

Q282. Answer: C

Explanation: The glucose tolerance test measures blood glucose levels over a 3-hour period. This allows evaluation of how the body processes glucose. Multiple readings improve diagnostic accuracy. Shorter tests are used for screening only. This test confirms gestational diabetes diagnosis. ##

Q283. Answer: B

Explanation: Elevated glucose levels lead to osmotic diuresis in the fetus. This increases urine production, resulting in polyhydramnios. Excess fluid accumulates in the amniotic sac. Other mechanisms do not significantly increase fluid volume. Monitoring is essential to manage complications. ##

Q284. Answer: C

Explanation: Fetal hyperinsulinemia persists after birth. Once maternal glucose supply is removed, insulin lowers blood glucose levels. This leads to hypoglycemia. Early feeding helps stabilize glucose levels. Monitoring is essential in neonatal care. Other factors do not explain this condition. ##

Q285. Answer: C

Explanation: Pharmacologic therapy is required when diet alone fails to control glucose levels. This ensures proper glycemic control. Monitoring helps guide therapy adjustments. Delaying intervention increases risks. Early management improves maternal and fetal outcomes. ##

Q286. Answer: A

Explanation: Macrosomia increases the risk of shoulder dystocia during delivery. The fetal shoulders may become impacted in the birth canal. This can lead to complications if not managed appropriately. Early identification helps plan delivery. Other options are not directly related. ##

Q287. Answer: D

Explanation: Gestational diabetes leads to both macrosomia and polyhydramnios. Elevated glucose affects fetal metabolism and fluid balance. These findings indicate metabolic imbalance. Early diagnosis allows appropriate intervention. Other conditions do not typically present this way. ##

Q288. Answer: A

Explanation: Women with gestational diabetes have an increased risk of developing type 2 diabetes later in life. This risk persists after pregnancy. Follow-up screening is essential. Lifestyle modifications can reduce progression. Other options are not primary long-term risks. ##

Q289. Answer: C
Explanation: Some newborns require minimal assistance during transition. Rapid improvement indicates mild adaptation difficulty. Initial weak responses are common. Recovery with simple interventions shows adequate physiological reserve. Monitoring ensures continued stability. This reflects a temporary adjustment phase. ##
Q290. Answer: D
Explanation: Poor glucose control leads to increased fetal urination and excessive growth. This results in polyhydramnios and macrosomia. These changes cause abdominal distension and breathing discomfort. The condition reflects metabolic imbalance. Early intervention is required to prevent complications. ##
Q291. Answer: D
Explanation: Elevated maternal glucose leads to increased fetal insulin production. Insulin promotes fat storage and tissue growth. This results in macrosomia. Other options do not explain this mechanism. Maintaining maternal glucose levels helps prevent excessive fetal growth. ##
Q292. Answer: D
Explanation: The glucose tolerance test measures blood glucose levels over a 3-hour period. This provides multiple readings to assess glucose metabolism. It confirms gestational diabetes diagnosis. Shorter tests are used for screening only. Accurate diagnosis guides appropriate management. ##
Q293. Answer: D
Explanation: Elevated glucose levels cause osmotic diuresis in the fetus. This increases urine production, leading to polyhydramnios. Excess fluid accumulates in the amniotic sac. Other processes do not significantly increase fluid volume. Monitoring helps detect and manage this condition. ##
Q294. Answer: B
Explanation: Fetal hyperinsulinemia persists after birth. When maternal glucose supply stops, insulin lowers blood glucose levels rapidly. This results in hypoglycemia. Early feeding helps stabilize levels. Monitoring is essential in neonatal care. Other factors do not explain this condition. ##
Q295. Answer: D
Explanation: Pharmacologic therapy is needed when diet alone fails to control glucose levels. This ensures proper glycemic control. Monitoring helps guide treatment adjustments. Delaying intervention increases risks. Early management improves outcomes for both mother and fetus. ##
Q296. Answer: B
Explanation: Patient identification is critical for safe medication administration. Failure to verify identity increases risk of harm. Reporting ensures accountability and adherence to standards. Following institutional policy is required. Ignoring the issue compromises patient safety. This action promotes quality care. ##
Q297. Answer: A
Explanation: Milk production depends on regular stimulation. Inconsistent pumping reduces prolactin levels. Maintaining frequent sessions helps restore supply. Consistent breast emptying supports ongoing production. Education encourages adherence to routine. This approach improves lactation outcomes. ##
Q298. Answer: B
Explanation: Women with gestational diabetes have a higher risk of developing type 2 diabetes later in life. This risk persists after pregnancy. Follow-up screening is essential for early detection. Lifestyle changes can reduce progression. Other options are not primary long-term risks. ##
Q299. Answer: A
Explanation: These signs indicate increased work of breathing. Decreased oxygen saturation confirms inadequate gas exchange. Persistent symptoms suggest respiratory distress. Immediate intervention is required. Monitoring guides treatment decisions. Early management improves neonatal outcomes. ##
Q300. Answer: B

Explanation: Poorly controlled diabetes leads to increased fetal urination and excessive growth. This results in polyhydramnios and macrosomia. These changes cause abdominal distension and breathing difficulty. The condition reflects metabolic imbalance. Early intervention is necessary to prevent complications. ## Question (301-400)

Question (301-400)

Q301. The first stage of labor ends with which event?
(A) Descent of fetal head
(B) Full cervical dilation
(C) Onset of contractions
(D) Rupture of membranes

Q302. Which intervention is commonly used to augment labor contractions?
(A) Insulin therapy
(B) Oxytocin infusion
(C) Antibiotic therapy
(D) Magnesium sulfate

Q303. Early decelerations during labor are most commonly associated with what cause?
(A) Uterine rupture
(B) Cord compression
(C) Head compression
(D) Placental insufficiency

Q304. The primary goal of pain management during labor is to achieve what outcome?
(A) Complete unconsciousness
(B) Delay of delivery process
(C) Pain relief with safety
(D) Elimination of contractions

Q305. A laboring patient has weak and irregular contractions with minimal cervical change. What is the most appropriate intervention?
(A) Encourage fluid restriction
(B) Initiate oxytocin infusion
(C) Delay further monitoring
(D) Stop labor assessment

Q306. A patient in labor receives epidural anesthesia. What effect should the nurse anticipate?
(A) Stronger contractions
(B) Increased pain sensation
(C) Reduced pain perception
(D) Faster cervical dilation

Q307. A laboring woman is being induced due to prolonged pregnancy. What is the primary purpose of induction?
(A) Stimulate uterine contractions
(B) Delay labor onset
(C) Prevent cervical dilation
(D) Reduce fetal growth

Q308. A patient is undergoing a trial of labor after cesarean (VBAC). What is the most serious complication to monitor for?
(A) Infection risk
(B) Slow contractions
(C) Uterine rupture
(D) Mild bleeding

Q309. A laboring patient is receiving oxytocin infusion. What is the priority nursing assessment?
(A) Evaluate dietary intake
(B) Assess skin condition

(C) Monitor contraction pattern
(D) Check urine color
Q310. A laboring woman suddenly experiences severe abdominal pain, loss of fetal station, and abnormal fetal heart rate after attempting VBAC. What is the most likely complication?
(A) Uterine rupture
(B) Shoulder dystocia
(C) Placental abruption
(D) Cord prolapse
Q311. The second stage of labor begins with which event?
(A) Rupture of membranes
(B) Placental separation
(C) Onset of contractions
(D) Full cervical dilation
Q312. Variable decelerations during labor are most commonly caused by what factor?
(A) Head compression
(B) Cord compression
(C) Uterine rupture
(D) Placental aging
Q313. Which method is commonly used for cervical ripening before labor induction?
(A) Diuretic medication use
(B) Insulin infusion therapy
(C) Antibiotic administration
(D) Prostaglandin administration
Q314. The third stage of labor ends with which event?
(A) Delivery of placenta
(B) Fetal descent completion
(C) Full cervical dilation
(D) Onset of contractions
Q315. A laboring patient shows inadequate contraction strength and slow cervical dilation. What is the most appropriate intervention?
(A) Start oxytocin infusion
(B) Delay further assessment
(C) Restrict oral fluids
(D) Stop fetal monitoring
Q316. A patient receiving epidural anesthesia experiences a drop in blood pressure. What is the priority nursing action?
(A) Delay intervention
(B) Restrict positioning
(C) Stop all monitoring
(D) Increase IV fluids
Q317. A laboring woman is undergoing induction with oxytocin. What is the primary goal of this therapy?
(A) Stimulate uterine contractions
(B) Delay cervical dilation
(C) Reduce fetal movement
(D) Prevent labor onset
Q318. A patient attempting VBAC is monitored closely during labor. Which sign indicates possible uterine rupture?

(A) Sudden severe pain
(B) Mild discomfort
(C) Gradual dilation
(D) Stable heart rate

Q319. A laboring patient receiving oxytocin develops frequent contractions with minimal relaxation time. What is the priority action?
(A) Encourage ambulation
(B) Increase medication dose
(C) Stop fetal monitoring
(D) Reduce oxytocin rate

Q320. A laboring woman suddenly experiences a gush of fluid followed by a visible umbilical cord at the vaginal opening and abnormal fetal heart rate. What is the most likely complication?
(A) Cord prolapse
(B) Shoulder dystocia
(C) Uterine rupture
(D) Placental abruption

Q321. The fourth stage of labor primarily involves what period?
(A) Placental separation process
(B) Fetal descent progression
(C) Immediate postpartum recovery
(D) Active cervical dilation phase

Q322. Late decelerations during labor are most commonly associated with what cause?
(A) Maternal position change
(B) Cord compression effect
(C) Placental insufficiency
(D) Head compression response

Q323. Vacuum-assisted delivery is indicated primarily for which purpose?
(A) Reduce uterine tone
(B) Assist fetal descent
(C) Delay delivery process
(D) Prevent contractions

Q324. Forceps delivery requires which essential condition before use?
(A) Early labor phase
(B) Fully dilated cervix
(C) Reduced contractions
(D) Intact membranes

Q325. A laboring patient has prolonged labor with minimal cervical change and adequate contractions. What is the most appropriate intervention?
(A) Assess for obstruction
(B) Encourage fluid restriction
(C) Increase oxytocin dose
(D) Delay further evaluation

Q326. A patient undergoing epidural analgesia reports dizziness and hypotension shortly after administration. What is the priority action?
(A) Encourage ambulation
(B) Delay monitoring
(C) Stop all interventions
(D) Increase IV fluid rate

Q327. A laboring woman receiving oxytocin develops contractions every minute lasting 90 seconds. What is the most appropriate action?
(A) Increase oxytocin dose
(B) Delay intervention
(C) Reduce or stop oxytocin
(D) Encourage ambulation
Q328. A patient attempting VBAC reports sudden sharp abdominal pain and abnormal fetal heart tracing. What is the most likely concern?
(A) Uterine rupture event
(B) Placental separation
(C) Shoulder dystocia event
(D) Cord prolapse condition
Q329. A laboring patient is being prepared for cesarean delivery due to fetal distress. What is the primary goal of this procedure?
(A) Reduce maternal contractions
(B) Prevent cervical dilation
(C) Rapid delivery of fetus
(D) Delay labor progression
Q330. A laboring woman suddenly reports intense abdominal pain followed by cessation of contractions, abnormal fetal heart rate, and loss of fetal station during active labor. What is the most likely diagnosis requiring immediate intervention?
(A) Placental abruption case
(B) Cord prolapse condition
(C) Uterine rupture emergency
(D) Shoulder dystocia event
Q331. The most effective pushing technique during the second stage of labor involves what action?
(A) Relaxing during contractions
(B) Holding breath continuously
(C) Bearing down with contractions
(D) Avoiding all movement
Q332. Internal fetal monitoring requires which condition before placement?
(A) Complete fetal descent
(B) Ruptured membranes
(C) Absence of contractions
(D) Full cervical dilation
Q333. The primary purpose of amniotomy during labor is to achieve what outcome?
(A) Enhance labor progress
(B) Delay contractions onset
(C) Prevent cervical dilation
(D) Reduce fetal movement
Q334. Shoulder dystocia occurs when which event happens during delivery?
(A) Umbilical cord descends
(B) Fetal shoulders impacted
(C) Placenta fails to detach
(D) Cervix fails to dilate
Q335. A laboring patient has prolonged second stage despite strong contractions and effective pushing efforts. What should be assessed next?
(A) Dietary intake pattern

(B) Frequency of contractions
(C) Fetal position and descent
(D) Maternal hydration status

Q336. A patient receiving epidural analgesia reports inability to feel contractions and has decreased urge to push. What is the most appropriate nursing response?
(A) Discontinue epidural immediately
(B) Encourage ambulation
(C) Provide coaching for pushing
(D) Delay further assessment

Q337. A laboring woman undergoing induction with oxytocin shows a normal contraction pattern and reassuring fetal heart tracing. What is the next nursing action?
(A) Delay further care
(B) Increase oxytocin dose
(C) Stop fetal monitoring
(D) Continue current management

Q338. A patient undergoing assisted delivery with vacuum extraction is at risk for which fetal complication?
(A) Scalp injury formation
(B) Uterine rupture event
(C) Umbilical cord compression
(D) Placental separation issue

Q339. A laboring patient experiences sudden fetal bradycardia following rupture of membranes. What is the priority assessment?
(A) Monitor contraction strength
(B) Check for cord prolapse
(C) Evaluate hydration status
(D) Assess maternal comfort

Q340. A laboring woman suddenly develops severe abdominal pain, vaginal bleeding, abnormal fetal heart rate, and loss of uterine tone during active labor following induction. What is the most likely complication requiring immediate intervention?
(A) Uterine rupture emergency
(B) Cord prolapse condition
(C) Shoulder dystocia event
(D) Normal labor variation

Q341. The latent phase of labor is characterized primarily by what feature?
(A) Slow cervical dilation
(B) Strong pushing efforts
(C) Placental separation
(D) Rapid fetal descent

Q342. Which intervention is commonly used to relieve pain without medication during labor?
(A) Breathing techniques
(B) Antibiotic therapy
(C) Insulin administration
(D) Fluid restriction

Q343. The active phase of labor is defined by which pattern?
(A) Minimal contraction activity
(B) Placental delivery process
(C) Rapid cervical dilation

(D) Fetal engagement only

Q344. Which position helps relieve cord compression during labor?

(A) Supine flat position
(B) Standing upright position
(C) Knee-chest position
(D) Semi-Fowler position

Q345. A laboring patient has adequate contractions but no cervical change for several hours. What should be evaluated first?

(A) Frequency of contractions
(B) Maternal dietary intake
(C) Fetal position and pelvis
(D) Urine output pattern

Q346. A patient receiving epidural analgesia develops urinary retention during labor. What is the most appropriate nursing action?

(A) Delay intervention
(B) Encourage fluid restriction
(C) Increase ambulation
(D) Insert urinary catheter

Q347. A laboring woman receiving oxytocin shows contractions every 3 minutes with reassuring fetal heart tracing. What is the appropriate action?

(A) Maintain current infusion rate
(B) Stop monitoring process
(C) Delay further assessment
(D) Increase oxytocin dose

Q348. A patient undergoing forceps delivery is at risk for which maternal complication?

(A) Placental insufficiency
(B) Uterine rupture
(C) Vaginal tissue injury
(D) Cord compression

Q349. A laboring patient experiences sudden fetal heart rate deceleration after epidural placement. What is the priority action?

(A) Stop monitoring
(B) Increase medication dose
(C) Reposition the patient
(D) Delay response

Q350. A laboring woman receiving induction develops severe abdominal pain, abnormal fetal heart tracing, and cessation of contractions shortly after oxytocin administration. What is the most likely complication requiring immediate intervention?

(A) Cord prolapse condition
(B) Shoulder dystocia event
(C) Uterine rupture emergency
(D) Normal labor progression

Q351. The transition phase of labor occurs near full dilation and is marked by strong contractions and increased maternal discomfort.

(A) Second stage phase
(B) Late first stage phase
(C) Fourth stage phase
(D) Third stage phase

Q352. Effacement refers to the thinning and shortening of the cervix as labor progresses toward delivery.
(A) Uterine contraction pattern
(B) Fetal descent movement
(C) Cervical thinning process
(D) Placental separation event
Q353. Which factor increases the likelihood of successful vaginal birth after cesarean (VBAC) in a laboring patient?
(A) Multiple uterine scars
(B) Induction with high dose
(C) Previous vaginal delivery
(D) Large fetal size
Q354. Which analgesic method provides continuous pain relief while allowing the patient to remain awake during labor?
(A) Sedative medication method
(B) Local infiltration method
(C) Epidural anesthesia method
(D) General anesthesia method
Q355. A laboring patient experiences strong contractions every 2 minutes with minimal cervical change over several hours. What should be assessed next to guide management?
(A) Maternal fluid intake
(B) Dietary intake pattern
(C) Fetal position alignment
(D) Frequency of contractions
Q356. A patient receiving epidural analgesia develops hypotension and fetal heart rate changes shortly after administration. What is the priority nursing intervention?
(A) Encourage ambulation
(B) Stop all monitoring
(C) Delay intervention
(D) Increase IV fluid rate
Q357. A laboring woman undergoing oxytocin induction develops frequent contractions with minimal relaxation time between them. What is the most appropriate action to ensure safety?
(A) Delay intervention
(B) Increase infusion rate
(C) Encourage ambulation
(D) Reduce or stop oxytocin
Q358. A patient undergoing vacuum-assisted delivery requires monitoring for which immediate neonatal finding after birth?
(A) Placental separation delay
(B) Scalp swelling or bruising
(C) Cord compression signs
(D) Uterine contraction pattern
Q359. A laboring patient experiences sudden fetal bradycardia following rupture of membranes during active labor. What is the priority nursing action to address this change?
(A) Evaluate contraction strength
(B) Assess for cord prolapse
(C) Delay immediate response
(D) Monitor maternal diet

Q360. A laboring woman receiving oxytocin suddenly develops severe abdominal pain, abnormal fetal heart tracing, cessation of contractions, and loss of fetal station during active labor. What is the most likely complication requiring emergency intervention?
(A) Shoulder dystocia event
(B) Uterine rupture emergency
(C) Normal labor variation
(D) Cord prolapse condition

Q361. The second stage of labor involves the period from full cervical dilation to delivery of the fetus with active maternal pushing.
(A) Expulsive phase process
(B) Latent phase process
(C) Placental phase process
(D) Recovery phase process

Q362. Station refers to the position of the fetal presenting part in relation to the maternal ischial spines during labor progress.
(A) Contraction intensity level
(B) Placental attachment level
(C) Fetal descent measurement
(D) Cervical dilation scale

Q363. Which factor is most important to assess before performing operative vaginal delivery using forceps or vacuum?
(A) Fetal head engagement
(B) Contraction frequency
(C) Maternal dietary intake
(D) Urine output pattern

Q364. Which method of pain relief provides rapid onset but shorter duration compared to epidural analgesia during labor?
(A) Intravenous opioid administration
(B) Continuous epidural infusion
(C) General anesthesia method
(D) Local anesthetic block

Q365. A laboring patient has strong contractions every 2-3 minutes but slow fetal descent despite full dilation. What should be assessed to guide further management?
(A) Fetal position alignment
(B) Dietary intake status
(C) Frequency of contractions
(D) Maternal hydration level

Q366. A patient receiving epidural analgesia experiences decreased blood pressure and changes in fetal heart rate. What is the priority intervention?
(A) Increase IV fluid administration
(B) Stop all monitoring processes
(C) Encourage immediate ambulation
(D) Delay intervention temporarily

Q367. A laboring woman receiving oxytocin develops contractions lasting 90 seconds with minimal relaxation between them. What is the most appropriate action?
(A) Increase infusion rate
(B) Decrease or stop oxytocin
(C) Delay immediate action

(D) Encourage ambulation

Q368. A patient undergoing vacuum-assisted delivery requires monitoring for which neonatal complication immediately after birth?

(A) Placental separation delay
(B) Scalp edema formation
(C) Uterine contraction issue
(D) Umbilical cord compression

Q369. A laboring patient develops sudden fetal bradycardia immediately after rupture of membranes during active labor. What is the priority nursing action to address this emergency?

(A) Delay further response
(B) Assess for cord prolapse
(C) Evaluate dietary intake
(D) Monitor contraction strength

Q370. A laboring woman receiving oxytocin develops sudden severe abdominal pain, cessation of contractions, abnormal fetal heart tracing, and loss of fetal station during active labor. What is the most likely diagnosis requiring immediate surgical intervention?

(A) Normal labor progression
(B) Shoulder dystocia event
(C) Cord prolapse condition
(D) Uterine rupture emergency

Q371. Engagement occurs when the widest diameter of the fetal head passes through the pelvic inlet during labor progression.

(A) Cervical dilation phase
(B) Fetal head entry stage
(C) Uterine contraction phase
(D) Placental separation stage

Q372. Lightening refers to the descent of the fetal presenting part into the maternal pelvis before the onset of labor.

(A) Fetal descent process
(B) Cervical thinning stage
(C) Placental detachment event
(D) Contraction strengthening phase

Q373. Which condition is required before performing an amniotomy during labor management?

(A) Absence of contractions
(B) Engaged fetal head
(C) Full cervical dilation
(D) Complete fetal descent

Q374. Which type of anesthesia provides complete loss of sensation and consciousness during obstetric procedures?

(A) Local anesthesia method
(B) General anesthesia method
(C) Epidural anesthesia method
(D) Regional block method

Q375. A laboring patient has effective contractions and full dilation but experiences prolonged pushing with minimal fetal descent. What should be evaluated to guide intervention?

(A) Fetal position and rotation
(B) Frequency of contractions
(C) Hydration status level

(D) Maternal dietary intake

Q376. A patient receiving epidural analgesia develops hypotension and decreased fetal heart rate variability. What is the priority intervention to stabilize the condition?

(A) Stop all monitoring immediately
(B) Increase IV fluid infusion
(C) Delay intervention briefly
(D) Encourage upright ambulation

Q377. A laboring woman receiving oxytocin develops uterine tachysystole with contractions every minute and prolonged duration. What is the most appropriate action?

(A) Delay response temporarily
(B) Encourage ambulation
(C) Increase infusion rate
(D) Reduce or discontinue oxytocin

Q378. A patient undergoing forceps-assisted delivery requires monitoring for which immediate maternal complication following the procedure?

(A) Uterine contraction delay
(B) Perineal tissue trauma
(C) Umbilical cord issue
(D) Placental insufficiency

Q379. A laboring patient develops sudden fetal bradycardia immediately after artificial rupture of membranes. What is the priority nursing action in this situation?

(A) Evaluate contraction strength
(B) Assess for cord prolapse
(C) Monitor dietary intake
(D) Delay immediate action

Q380. A laboring woman undergoing augmentation with oxytocin suddenly reports severe abdominal pain, cessation of contractions, abnormal fetal heart tracing, and palpable fetal parts through the abdomen. What is the most likely complication requiring emergency intervention?

(A) Normal labor variation
(B) Uterine rupture emergency
(C) Cord prolapse condition
(D) Shoulder dystocia event

Q381. Crowning occurs when the fetal head remains visible at the vaginal opening without receding between contractions during birth.

(A) Uterine relaxation phase
(B) Early dilation phase
(C) Placental separation stage
(D) Final expulsion stage

Q382. The Ferguson reflex stimulates increased uterine contractions in response to pressure from the fetal presenting part on the cervix.

(A) Neurohormonal contraction response
(B) Placental blood flow mechanism
(C) Fetal oxygen exchange process
(D) Cervical dilation measurement

Q383. Which condition increases the risk of shoulder dystocia during vaginal delivery of the fetus?

(A) Reduced maternal age
(B) Early membrane rupture
(C) Frequent contractions

(D) Large fetal size

Q384. Which pharmacologic method is commonly used to induce labor by stimulating uterine contractions effectively?

(A) Insulin infusion therapy
(B) Diuretic drug therapy
(C) Oxytocin administration
(D) Antibiotic medication use

Q385. A laboring patient has strong contractions but minimal fetal descent despite full cervical dilation and adequate pushing efforts. What should be evaluated next to guide intervention?

(A) Maternal dietary intake
(B) Frequency of contractions
(C) Fetal head position
(D) Hydration status level

Q386. A patient receiving epidural analgesia develops hypotension with associated fetal heart rate changes shortly after placement. What is the priority nursing intervention to stabilize both mother and fetus?

(A) Delay intervention
(B) Encourage ambulation
(C) Increase IV fluid rate
(D) Stop all monitoring

Q387. A laboring woman undergoing oxytocin augmentation develops contractions every minute lasting over 90 seconds with minimal resting tone. What is the most appropriate action to ensure safety?

(A) Encourage ambulation
(B) Delay response
(C) Increase infusion rate
(D) Discontinue oxytocin infusion

Q388. A patient undergoing vacuum-assisted delivery requires monitoring for which neonatal complication immediately following birth?

(A) Scalp swelling formation
(B) Uterine contraction issue
(C) Placental separation delay
(D) Umbilical cord compression

Q389. A laboring patient experiences sudden fetal bradycardia immediately after artificial rupture of membranes, with no improvement after repositioning. What is the priority next action?

(A) Monitor maternal diet
(B) Perform immediate cord assessment
(C) Delay further action
(D) Evaluate contraction pattern

Q390. A laboring woman receiving high-dose oxytocin develops sudden severe abdominal pain, cessation of contractions, vaginal bleeding, abnormal fetal heart tracing, and easily palpable fetal parts through the abdomen. What is the most likely diagnosis requiring emergency surgical intervention?

(A) Cord prolapse condition
(B) Uterine rupture emergency
(C) Normal labor progression
(D) Shoulder dystocia event

Q391. The mechanism of labor includes cardinal movements that allow the fetus to adapt and pass through the maternal pelvis during delivery.
(A) Sequential positional changes
(B) Uterine contraction cycle
(C) Placental attachment process
(D) Cervical effacement phase
Q392. Flexion during labor refers to the movement that allows the fetal chin to move toward the chest, reducing the presenting diameter.
(A) Placental detachment phase
(B) Uterine contraction pattern
(C) Head bending movement
(D) Pelvic expansion process
Q393. Which condition is required before performing vacuum-assisted delivery during the second stage of labor?
(A) Intact membranes
(B) Weak contractions
(C) Fully dilated cervix
(D) Early labor phase
Q394. Which medication is commonly used for pain relief during labor while maintaining maternal awareness and participation?
(A) Deep sedation method
(B) Complete nerve block
(C) Epidural analgesia
(D) General anesthesia
Q395. A laboring patient has prolonged labor with adequate contractions but minimal cervical change. What should be evaluated to determine the underlying cause?
(A) Maternal dietary intake
(B) Pelvic adequacy and fetal position
(C) Urine output level
(D) Frequency of contractions
Q396. A patient receiving epidural anesthesia develops hypotension and decreased fetal heart rate shortly after administration. What is the priority intervention to stabilize the condition?
(A) Encourage ambulation
(B) Delay intervention
(C) Stop all monitoring
(D) Increase IV fluid infusion
Q397. A laboring woman receiving oxytocin develops uterine tachysystole with contractions every minute and prolonged duration. What is the most appropriate action to prevent fetal compromise?
(A) Encourage ambulation
(B) Discontinue oxytocin infusion
(C) Increase infusion rate
(D) Delay response
Q398. A patient undergoing forceps-assisted delivery requires monitoring for which immediate maternal complication after the procedure?
(A) Umbilical cord compression
(B) Uterine contraction delay
(C) Vaginal tissue trauma
(D) Placental insufficiency

Q399. A laboring patient develops sudden fetal bradycardia immediately after artificial rupture of membranes and does not improve with repositioning. What is the priority next step in management?
(A) Delay further action
(B) Monitor maternal diet
(C) Evaluate contraction pattern
(D) Perform immediate cord assessment

Q400. A laboring woman receiving oxytocin develops sudden severe abdominal pain, vaginal bleeding, abnormal fetal heart tracing, cessation of contractions, and easily palpable fetal parts during active labor. What is the most likely diagnosis requiring emergency intervention?
(A) Normal labor variation
(B) Cord prolapse condition
(C) Uterine rupture emergency
(D) Shoulder dystocia event

Answer Key and Explanation (301-400)

Q301. Answer: B
Explanation: The first stage of labor begins with regular contractions and ends when the cervix is fully dilated to 10 cm. This allows the fetus to pass into the birth canal. Other events may occur during labor but do not define the end of this stage. Proper assessment of dilation is essential. This stage prepares for delivery. ##

Q302. Answer: B
Explanation: Oxytocin is used to stimulate uterine contractions and enhance labor progress. It is commonly used for augmentation when contractions are inadequate. Careful monitoring is required to avoid complications. Other medications do not have this effect. Proper dosing ensures safe labor progression. ##

Q303. Answer: C
Explanation: Early decelerations are caused by fetal head compression during contractions. This leads to a vagal response and temporary decrease in heart rate. It is usually benign and expected during labor. Other causes are associated with different patterns. Monitoring ensures fetal well-being. ##

Q304. Answer: C
Explanation: Pain management aims to relieve discomfort while maintaining maternal and fetal safety. It should not interfere with labor progression. Various methods are used depending on patient needs. Monitoring ensures effectiveness and safety. Other options are not appropriate goals. ##

Q305. Answer: B
Explanation: Weak and ineffective contractions may require augmentation with oxytocin. This helps improve contraction strength and frequency. Proper monitoring ensures safe administration. Delaying intervention may prolong labor. Early management supports labor progression. ##

Q306. Answer: C
Explanation: Epidural anesthesia reduces pain by blocking nerve signals from the lower body. It provides effective pain relief during labor. Monitoring is required for potential side effects. It does not directly increase contractions or speed dilation. Proper care ensures maternal comfort and safety. ##

Q307. Answer: A
Explanation: Induction is performed to initiate labor by stimulating uterine contractions. It is used when continuation of pregnancy poses risks. Methods include medications and mechanical techniques. Monitoring ensures effectiveness and safety. Other options do not reflect the purpose of induction. ##

Q308. Answer: C
Explanation: Uterine rupture is the most serious complication during VBAC. It occurs when the previous uterine scar opens during labor. This can lead to severe maternal and fetal complications. Continuous monitoring is essential. Early detection allows immediate intervention. ##

Q309. Answer: C
Explanation: Monitoring contraction frequency, duration, and intensity is essential during oxytocin infusion. Excessive contractions can compromise fetal oxygenation. Continuous assessment helps prevent complications. Other assessments are less critical in this context. Proper monitoring ensures safe labor progression. ##

Q310. Answer: A
Explanation: Sudden severe pain, loss of fetal station, and abnormal fetal heart rate are classic signs of uterine rupture. This is a life-threatening emergency. Immediate intervention is required to protect both mother and fetus. VBAC increases this risk. Rapid recognition improves outcomes. ##

Q311. Answer: D

Explanation: The second stage of labor begins when the cervix is fully dilated to 10 cm. This stage continues until the delivery of the fetus. It involves active pushing efforts by the mother. Other events occur at different stages. Proper identification helps guide care during delivery. ##

Q312. Answer: B

Explanation: Variable decelerations are caused by umbilical cord compression. This leads to abrupt decreases in fetal heart rate. The pattern can vary in timing and shape. Interventions focus on relieving pressure on the cord. Other causes produce different deceleration patterns. ##

Q313. Answer: D

Explanation: Prostaglandins are used to soften and dilate the cervix before induction. This improves the success of labor induction. They prepare the cervix for contractions. Other medications do not have this effect. Proper use enhances labor progression. ##

Q314. Answer: A

Explanation: The third stage of labor begins after delivery of the fetus and ends with delivery of the placenta. This stage involves placental separation and expulsion. Proper management reduces bleeding risks. Other events occur in earlier stages. Monitoring ensures safe completion. ##

Q315. Answer: A

Explanation: Inadequate contractions can be improved with oxytocin infusion. This helps increase contraction strength and frequency. Proper monitoring ensures safe administration. Delaying intervention may prolong labor. Effective management supports labor progression. ##

Q316. Answer: D

Explanation: Epidural anesthesia can cause hypotension due to vasodilation. Increasing IV fluids helps improve blood pressure. Monitoring maternal and fetal status is essential. Positioning may also be adjusted. Prompt intervention prevents complications. ##

Q317. Answer: A

Explanation: Oxytocin is used to stimulate uterine contractions for induction or augmentation. It helps initiate or strengthen labor. Careful monitoring is required to avoid excessive contractions. Proper dosing ensures effectiveness. Other options do not reflect its purpose. ##

Q318. Answer: A

Explanation: Sudden severe abdominal pain is a key sign of uterine rupture. It may be accompanied by fetal distress and loss of fetal station. This is a medical emergency. Immediate intervention is required. Early recognition improves outcomes. ##

Q319. Answer: D

Explanation: Excessive contractions can reduce fetal oxygenation. Reducing or stopping oxytocin helps restore normal contraction patterns. Continuous monitoring is essential. Prompt action prevents complications. Other options may worsen the condition. ##

Q320. Answer: A

Explanation: Cord prolapse occurs when the umbilical cord descends ahead of the fetus. This can compress the cord and compromise fetal oxygenation. It is a medical emergency. Immediate intervention is required. Early recognition improves fetal outcomes. ##

Q321. Answer: C

Explanation: The fourth stage of labor refers to the immediate postpartum recovery period. It typically lasts 1-2 hours after delivery. During this time, the mother is monitored for bleeding and stabilization. Uterine contraction and vital signs are closely assessed. Other options describe earlier stages of labor. ##

Q322. Answer: C

Explanation: Late decelerations occur due to uteroplacental insufficiency. This results in decreased oxygen delivery to the fetus during contractions. It is a concerning pattern requiring intervention. Other causes produce different deceleration types. Prompt recognition helps prevent fetal compromise. ##

Q323. Answer: B

Explanation: Vacuum-assisted delivery is used to help guide the fetus through the birth canal. It is indicated when labor is prolonged or maternal effort is insufficient. It assists fetal descent during the second stage. Proper use reduces delivery complications. Other options are not indications. ##

Q324. Answer: B

Explanation: Forceps delivery requires full cervical dilation to prevent injury. The fetal head must also be engaged. This ensures safe application of the instrument. Other conditions are not appropriate for forceps use. Proper criteria reduce complications during assisted delivery. ##

Q325. Answer: A

Explanation: Prolonged labor despite adequate contractions suggests possible obstruction. Assessment of fetal position and pelvic adequacy is necessary. Increasing oxytocin may not help if obstruction exists. Early evaluation prevents complications. Proper diagnosis guides management decisions. ##

Q326. Answer: D

Explanation: Epidural analgesia can cause vasodilation leading to hypotension. Increasing IV fluids helps restore blood pressure. Monitoring maternal and fetal status is essential. Positioning adjustments may also help. Prompt intervention prevents complications such as fetal distress. ##

Q327. Answer: C

Explanation: Excessive contractions reduce uterine relaxation time and impair fetal oxygenation. Reducing or stopping oxytocin helps normalize contraction patterns. Continuous monitoring is essential. Prompt action prevents fetal distress. Other options may worsen the condition. ##

Q328. Answer: A

Explanation: Sudden sharp abdominal pain with fetal distress suggests uterine rupture. This is a serious complication during VBAC. Immediate intervention is required. Delay can lead to severe maternal and fetal outcomes. Continuous monitoring helps early detection. ##

Q329. Answer: C

Explanation: Cesarean delivery is performed to rapidly deliver the fetus when vaginal delivery is unsafe. It is commonly indicated in fetal distress. The goal is to prevent further compromise. Timely intervention improves outcomes. Other options do not reflect the purpose of the procedure. ##

Q330. Answer: C

Explanation: Sudden severe pain, cessation of contractions, and loss of fetal station are classic signs of uterine rupture. This is a life-threatening emergency. Immediate surgical intervention is required. Fetal distress is commonly present. Early recognition improves survival outcomes. Delay increases risk of severe complications. ##

Q331. Answer: C

Explanation: Effective pushing occurs when the mother bears down during contractions. This increases intra-abdominal pressure and aids fetal descent. Coordinating pushing with contractions maximizes efficiency. Relaxation occurs between contractions. Other options do not support delivery progress. Proper coaching improves outcomes. ##

Q332. Answer: B

Explanation: Internal fetal monitoring requires ruptured membranes to allow placement of the electrode. This provides direct measurement of fetal heart rate. It is more accurate than external monitoring. Other conditions are not required. Proper placement ensures reliable assessment. ##

Q333. Answer: A

Explanation: Amniotomy involves artificial rupture of membranes to stimulate labor. It increases prostaglandin release and strengthens contractions. This helps progress labor. It may also allow internal monitoring. Other options are not purposes of this procedure. ##

Q334. Answer: B

Explanation: Shoulder dystocia occurs when the fetal shoulders become stuck after the head is delivered. This prevents completion of delivery. It is an obstetric emergency requiring immediate intervention. Other options describe different complications. Prompt action reduces risk of injury. ##

Q335. Answer: C

Explanation: Prolonged second stage with adequate contractions suggests possible malposition or descent issue. Assessing fetal position helps determine the cause. This guides appropriate intervention such as repositioning or assisted delivery. Other factors are less critical. Early assessment prevents complications. ##

Q336. Answer: C

Explanation: Epidural analgesia reduces sensation, including the urge to push. The nurse should provide guidance and coaching during contractions. This helps maintain effective pushing efforts. Discontinuing epidural is not usually necessary. Continuous support improves labor outcomes. ##

Q337. Answer: D

Explanation: When contractions and fetal status are normal, the current management should be continued. Increasing oxytocin is unnecessary and may cause complications. Continuous monitoring ensures ongoing safety. Stable conditions indicate effective treatment. Maintaining balance prevents adverse outcomes. ##

Q338. Answer: A

Explanation: Vacuum extraction can cause scalp injuries such as bruising or swelling. These are usually temporary but require monitoring. Proper technique reduces risk. Other complications are not directly related. Assessment of the newborn is essential after delivery. ##

Q339. Answer: B

Explanation: Sudden fetal bradycardia after membrane rupture suggests possible cord prolapse. Immediate assessment is required to confirm. This is an emergency requiring rapid intervention. Early detection improves fetal outcomes. Other assessments are secondary. ##

Q340. Answer: A

Explanation: Severe abdominal pain, bleeding, abnormal fetal heart rate, and loss of uterine tone indicate uterine rupture. This is a life-threatening emergency. Immediate surgical intervention is required. Delay increases risk of maternal and fetal death. Early recognition is critical. Rapid response improves survival outcomes. ##

Q341. Answer: A

Explanation: The latent phase is the early part of the first stage of labor. It involves slow cervical dilation and mild contractions. This phase prepares the cervix for active labor. Contractions gradually become stronger and more regular. Other options describe later stages of labor. ##

Q342. Answer: A

Explanation: Breathing techniques are non-pharmacologic methods used for pain relief during labor. They help the patient relax and manage contractions. These techniques reduce anxiety and improve coping. They are safe and commonly taught in childbirth education. Other options are not pain relief methods. ##

Q343. Answer: C

Explanation: The active phase involves rapid cervical dilation and stronger contractions. It follows the latent phase and progresses toward full dilation. Contractions become more regular and intense. This phase requires close monitoring. Other options do not define the active phase. ##

Q344. Answer: C

Explanation: The knee-chest position helps relieve pressure on the umbilical cord. It improves blood flow to the fetus during cord compression. This position is used in emergencies such as cord prolapse. Other positions may not be effective. Prompt positioning improves fetal oxygenation. ##

Q345. Answer: C

Explanation: Lack of cervical change despite adequate contractions suggests possible mechanical issues. Assessing fetal position and pelvic adequacy is essential. Malposition can delay labor progress. Identifying the cause guides further management. Other factors are less directly related. ##

Q346. Answer: D

Explanation: Epidural anesthesia can reduce bladder sensation, leading to urinary retention. Insertion of a catheter helps prevent bladder distension. Monitoring urine output is important. Early management prevents complications. Other options do not address the issue effectively. ##

Q347. Answer: A

Explanation: A contraction pattern every 2-3 minutes with reassuring fetal status is appropriate. The current oxytocin rate should be maintained. Increasing the dose is unnecessary and may cause complications. Continuous monitoring ensures safety. Stable patterns indicate effective management. ##

Q348. Answer: C

Explanation: Forceps delivery can cause vaginal or perineal tissue injury. Proper technique reduces risk but does not eliminate it. Monitoring for bleeding and trauma is essential. Other complications are less directly associated. Careful assessment ensures maternal safety. ##

Q349. Answer: C

Explanation: Repositioning the patient can improve uterine blood flow and fetal oxygenation. Epidural anesthesia may cause hypotension affecting the fetus. Immediate intervention is necessary. Monitoring ensures response effectiveness. Other options are inappropriate in this situation. ##

Q350. Answer: C

Explanation: Severe pain, abnormal fetal heart rate, and cessation of contractions suggest uterine rupture. This is a life-threatening emergency. It can occur with excessive uterine stimulation. Immediate surgical intervention is required. Early recognition improves maternal and fetal outcomes. Delay increases risk of severe complications. ##

Q351. Answer: B

Explanation: The transition phase is the final part of the first stage of labor. It occurs as the cervix dilates from 8 to 10 cm. Contractions become strong, frequent, and intense. Maternal discomfort and pressure increase significantly. Other stages involve different labor events. ##

Q352. Answer: C

Explanation: Effacement describes the thinning and shortening of the cervix in preparation for birth. It is measured in percentages from 0 to 100%. This process allows dilation to occur more effectively. It happens alongside cervical dilation. Other options describe different labor processes. ##

Q353. Answer: C

Explanation: A previous vaginal delivery increases the chance of successful VBAC. It indicates the pelvis can accommodate delivery. Multiple scars and large fetal size increase risk of complications. High-dose induction may increase rupture risk. Proper selection improves outcomes. ##

Q354. Answer: C

Explanation: Epidural anesthesia provides continuous pain relief while maintaining consciousness. It blocks nerve impulses from the lower body. It allows participation in labor while reducing pain. Monitoring is required for side effects. Other methods do not provide continuous controlled relief. ##

Q355. Answer: C

Explanation: Strong contractions with little progress suggest possible malposition. Assessing fetal position helps identify obstruction or alignment issues. This guides interventions such as repositioning. Other factors are less directly related. Early evaluation prevents prolonged labor complications. ##

Q356. Answer: D

Explanation: Epidural anesthesia can cause vasodilation leading to hypotension. Increasing IV fluids helps restore blood pressure. This improves uteroplacental perfusion. Monitoring fetal heart rate is essential. Prompt intervention prevents fetal compromise. ##

Q357. Answer: D
Explanation: Excessive contractions reduce uterine blood flow and fetal oxygenation. Reducing or stopping oxytocin helps restore normal patterns. Continuous monitoring is essential. Prompt action prevents fetal distress. Other options may worsen the situation. ##
Q358. Answer: B
Explanation: Vacuum-assisted delivery can cause scalp injuries such as bruising or swelling. These are usually temporary but require monitoring. Proper technique reduces risk. Newborn assessment is essential after delivery. Other options are not directly related to this procedure. ##
Q359. Answer: B
Explanation: Sudden fetal bradycardia after membrane rupture suggests cord prolapse. Immediate assessment is critical. This condition compromises fetal oxygenation. Rapid intervention improves outcomes. Other actions are secondary. Prompt recognition is essential. ##
Q360. Answer: B
Explanation: Severe pain, abnormal fetal tracing, and loss of station indicate uterine rupture. This is a life-threatening emergency. It may occur with excessive uterine stimulation. Immediate surgical intervention is required. Delay increases risk of maternal and fetal mortality. Early recognition improves outcomes. ##
Q361. Answer: A
Explanation: The second stage of labor begins at full cervical dilation and ends with delivery of the fetus. It is characterized by active maternal pushing and fetal descent. This stage requires coordination between contractions and pushing. Other phases refer to different stages of labor. Proper support improves delivery outcomes. ##
Q362. Answer: C
Explanation: Station measures the descent of the fetal presenting part relative to the ischial spines. It is expressed in negative and positive numbers. Zero station indicates alignment with the spines. This helps assess labor progress. Other options describe unrelated parameters. ##
Q363. Answer: A
Explanation: Operative vaginal delivery requires that the fetal head is engaged in the pelvis. This ensures safe application of instruments. Lack of engagement increases risk of injury. Other factors are less critical for this decision. Proper assessment reduces complications. ##
Q364. Answer: A
Explanation: Intravenous opioids provide rapid pain relief but have a shorter duration compared to epidural analgesia. They are useful for temporary pain control. However, they may affect maternal alertness. Epidurals provide longer-lasting relief. Choice depends on labor stage and patient needs. ##
Q365. Answer: A
Explanation: Strong contractions with slow descent suggest malposition of the fetus. Assessing fetal position helps identify issues such as occiput posterior position. This guides interventions like repositioning or assisted delivery. Other factors are less directly related. Early assessment improves outcomes. ##
Q366. Answer: A
Explanation: Epidural anesthesia can cause vasodilation leading to hypotension. Increasing IV fluids helps restore blood pressure. This improves uteroplacental perfusion. Monitoring fetal heart rate is essential. Prompt intervention prevents fetal compromise. Other actions are not appropriate initially. ##
Q367. Answer: B
Explanation: Excessive contraction duration reduces uterine blood flow and fetal oxygenation. Reducing or stopping oxytocin helps restore normal contraction patterns. Continuous monitoring is essential. Prompt action prevents fetal distress. Other options may worsen the condition. ##
Q368. Answer: B

Explanation: Vacuum extraction can cause scalp edema or bruising in the newborn. These findings are usually temporary but require monitoring. Proper technique reduces risk. Immediate newborn assessment is essential. Other options are not directly related to this procedure. ##

Q369. Answer: B

Explanation: Sudden fetal bradycardia after membrane rupture suggests cord prolapse. Immediate assessment is critical to confirm the condition. Cord compression reduces fetal oxygenation. Rapid intervention improves outcomes. Other actions are secondary. Prompt recognition is essential. ##

Q370. Answer: D

Explanation: Sudden severe pain, loss of contractions, and fetal distress indicate uterine rupture. This is a life-threatening emergency. It may occur with excessive uterine stimulation or prior uterine scar. Immediate surgical intervention is required. Delay increases risk of maternal and fetal mortality. Early recognition improves outcomes. ##

Q371. Answer: B

Explanation: Engagement refers to the passage of the fetal head into the pelvic inlet. It indicates that the presenting part has entered the true pelvis. This is an important milestone in labor progress. It is assessed using station measurements. Other options describe unrelated processes. ##

Q372. Answer: A

Explanation: Lightening occurs when the fetus moves downward into the pelvis. This often happens in late pregnancy before labor begins. It may relieve pressure on the diaphragm. However, it increases pelvic pressure. Other options describe different labor-related processes. ##

Q373. Answer: B

Explanation: Amniotomy should only be performed when the fetal head is engaged. This reduces the risk of cord prolapse. The procedure helps stimulate labor progression. Other conditions are not required. Proper assessment ensures safety during intervention. ##

Q374. Answer: B

Explanation: General anesthesia causes complete unconsciousness and loss of sensation. It is used for emergency procedures when rapid intervention is needed. It affects both maternal and fetal physiology. Epidural and local methods allow the patient to remain awake. Proper use ensures safety during surgery. ##

Q375. Answer: A

Explanation: Prolonged pushing with minimal descent suggests malposition or rotation issues. Assessing fetal position helps identify problems such as occiput posterior. This guides interventions like repositioning or assisted delivery. Other factors are less directly related. Early evaluation improves outcomes. ##

Q376. Answer: B

Explanation: Epidural analgesia can cause vasodilation leading to hypotension. Increasing IV fluids helps restore blood pressure. This improves uteroplacental perfusion and fetal status. Continuous monitoring is essential. Prompt action prevents complications. Other options are not appropriate initially. ##

Q377. Answer: D

Explanation: Uterine tachysystole reduces uterine relaxation time and fetal oxygenation. Reducing or stopping oxytocin helps normalize contraction patterns. Continuous monitoring is essential. Prompt intervention prevents fetal distress. Other actions may worsen the situation. ##

Q378. Answer: B

Explanation: Forceps delivery can cause perineal or vaginal trauma. Monitoring for bleeding and tissue injury is essential. Proper technique reduces risk but does not eliminate it. Early detection allows prompt management. Other complications are less directly related. ##

Q379. Answer: B

Explanation: Sudden fetal bradycardia after amniotomy suggests cord prolapse. Immediate assessment is required to confirm. Cord compression reduces fetal oxygenation. Rapid intervention improves outcomes. Other actions are secondary. Prompt recognition is critical in emergencies. ##

Q380. Answer: B

Explanation: Severe abdominal pain, cessation of contractions, and abnormal fetal tracing indicate uterine rupture. Palpable fetal parts confirm disruption of the uterine wall. This is a life-threatening emergency. Immediate surgical intervention is required. Delay increases risk of maternal and fetal death. Early recognition improves outcomes. ##

Q381. Answer: D

Explanation: Crowning is a key event in the second stage of labor when the fetal head stays visible. It indicates imminent delivery of the fetus. This occurs due to sustained descent and stretching of tissues. Proper support helps prevent perineal trauma. Other options describe unrelated phases. ##

Q382. Answer: A

Explanation: The Ferguson reflex is triggered by pressure on the cervix. This leads to oxytocin release and stronger uterine contractions. It plays a role in advancing labor. This reflex supports the progression toward delivery. Other options describe different physiological processes. ##

Q383. Answer: D

Explanation: A large fetal size increases the risk of shoulder dystocia. The shoulders may become impacted after delivery of the head. This creates difficulty in completing delivery. Early recognition allows prompt intervention. Other factors are less strongly associated. ##

Q384. Answer: C

Explanation: Oxytocin is widely used to induce labor by stimulating uterine contractions. It enhances contraction strength and frequency. Careful monitoring is required to prevent complications. It is a standard method in labor management. Other medications do not induce labor contractions. ##

Q385. Answer: C

Explanation: Strong contractions with minimal descent suggest possible malposition. Assessing fetal head position helps identify issues such as occiput posterior. This guides repositioning or assisted delivery. Other factors are less directly related. Early intervention improves outcomes. ##

Q386. Answer: C

Explanation: Epidural anesthesia can cause vasodilation leading to hypotension. Increasing IV fluids helps restore blood pressure. This improves uteroplacental perfusion and fetal status. Continuous monitoring is essential. Prompt action prevents complications. Other options are not appropriate initially. ##

Q387. Answer: D

Explanation: Excessive contractions reduce uterine relaxation time and fetal oxygenation. Discontinuing oxytocin helps normalize contraction patterns. Continuous monitoring is essential. Prompt intervention prevents fetal distress. Other actions may worsen the situation. ##

Q388. Answer: A

Explanation: Vacuum extraction can cause scalp swelling or bruising in the newborn. These findings are usually temporary but require observation. Proper technique reduces risk. Newborn assessment is essential after delivery. Other options are not directly related. ##

Q389. Answer: B

Explanation: Persistent fetal bradycardia after membrane rupture suggests cord prolapse. Immediate assessment is critical. Cord compression compromises fetal oxygenation. Rapid intervention improves outcomes. Other actions are secondary. Prompt recognition is essential in emergencies. ##

Q390. Answer: B

Explanation: Severe abdominal pain, bleeding, and abnormal fetal tracing indicate uterine rupture. Palpable fetal parts confirm disruption of the uterine wall. This is a life-threatening emergency.

Immediate surgical intervention is required. Delay increases risk of maternal and fetal death. Early recognition improves outcomes significantly. ##

Q391. Answer: A

Explanation: The cardinal movements describe the positional changes the fetus undergoes during labor. These include engagement, descent, flexion, and rotation. They help the fetus navigate the maternal pelvis. Proper progression ensures safe delivery. Other options describe unrelated processes. ##

Q392. Answer: C

Explanation: Flexion reduces the fetal head diameter by bringing the chin to the chest. This allows easier passage through the pelvis. It is an important cardinal movement of labor. Proper flexion supports efficient delivery. Other options are unrelated to this mechanism. ##

Q393. Answer: C

Explanation: Vacuum-assisted delivery requires full cervical dilation. This ensures safe application of the device. The fetal head must also be engaged. Performing it earlier increases risk of injury. Proper criteria reduce complications. Other options are not appropriate requirements. ##

Q394. Answer: C

Explanation: Epidural analgesia provides effective pain relief while allowing the patient to remain awake. It blocks nerve transmission from the lower body. It is widely used in labor management. Monitoring is required for side effects. Other methods may impair consciousness. ##

Q395. Answer: B

Explanation: Prolonged labor despite adequate contractions suggests possible obstruction. Assessing pelvic adequacy and fetal position is essential. Malposition or mismatch can delay progress. Early identification guides intervention. Other factors are less directly related. ##

Q396. Answer: D

Explanation: Epidural anesthesia causes vasodilation leading to hypotension. Increasing IV fluids helps restore blood pressure. This improves uteroplacental perfusion. Monitoring fetal status is essential. Prompt action prevents fetal compromise. Other options are inappropriate initially. ##

Q397. Answer: B

Explanation: Uterine tachysystole reduces relaxation time and fetal oxygenation. Stopping oxytocin helps restore normal contraction patterns. Continuous monitoring is essential. Prompt intervention prevents complications. Other actions may worsen the condition. ##

Q398. Answer: C

Explanation: Forceps delivery can cause vaginal or perineal trauma. Monitoring for bleeding and injury is essential. Proper technique reduces risk. Early detection allows prompt management. Other complications are less directly related. ##

Q399. Answer: D

Explanation: Persistent fetal bradycardia after membrane rupture suggests cord prolapse. Immediate assessment is critical. Cord compression compromises fetal oxygenation. Rapid intervention improves outcomes. Other actions are secondary. Prompt recognition is essential in emergencies. ##

Q400. Answer: C

Explanation: Severe pain, bleeding, and abnormal fetal tracing indicate uterine rupture. Palpable fetal parts confirm uterine wall disruption. This is a life-threatening emergency. Immediate surgical intervention is required. Delay increases risk of maternal and fetal mortality. Early recognition improves outcomes significantly. ## Question (401-500)

Question (401-500)

Q401. Extension during labor occurs when the fetal head moves upward under the pubic bone as it emerges from the birth canal.
(A) Head extension movement
(B) Pelvic widening process
(C) Placental separation stage
(D) Cervical dilation phase

Q402. External rotation occurs after delivery of the fetal head as it realigns with the shoulders to complete the birthing process.
(A) Uterine contraction pattern
(B) Cervical thinning process
(C) Shoulder alignment movement
(D) Placental detachment phase

Q403. Which condition must be confirmed before attempting a vaginal birth after cesarean (VBAC) to reduce complications?
(A) Previous uterine incision type
(B) Frequency of contractions
(C) Urine output level
(D) Maternal dietary intake

Q404. Which method is commonly used to monitor uterine contraction intensity internally during labor management?
(A) Fetal scalp electrode
(B) Intrauterine pressure catheter
(C) External ultrasound device
(D) Doppler monitoring device

Q405. A laboring patient has adequate contractions but failure of fetal descent during the second stage despite full dilation. What should be assessed next to determine management?
(A) Maternal dietary intake
(B) Frequency of contractions
(C) Urine output pattern
(D) Fetal position and pelvic fit

Q406. A patient receiving epidural analgesia develops hypotension with associated fetal heart rate decelerations shortly after placement. What is the priority intervention?
(A) Encourage ambulation
(B) Delay intervention
(C) Stop all monitoring immediately
(D) Increase IV fluid administration

Q407. A laboring woman receiving oxytocin develops uterine tachysystole with minimal resting tone between contractions. What is the most appropriate action to prevent fetal compromise?
(A) Increase infusion rate
(B) Delay response
(C) Encourage ambulation
(D) Discontinue oxytocin infusion

Q408. A postpartum patient is instructed on warning signs of complications; which symptom should be reported immediately?
(A) Occasional mood swings
(B) Breast fullness sensation

(C) Blurred vision episodes
(D) Mild fatigue feeling
Q409. A laboring patient develops sudden fetal bradycardia immediately after rupture of membranes that does not improve with repositioning. What is the priority next step in management?
(A) Evaluate contraction strength
(B) Assess for cord prolapse
(C) Delay further action
(D) Monitor maternal diet
Q410. A laboring woman receiving oxytocin develops sudden severe abdominal pain, vaginal bleeding, cessation of contractions, abnormal fetal heart tracing, and palpable fetal parts during active labor. What is the most likely complication requiring emergency surgical intervention?
(A) Cord prolapse condition
(B) Normal labor variation
(C) Shoulder dystocia event
(D) Uterine rupture emergency
Q411. Restitution occurs after delivery of the fetal head when it rotates to align with the shoulders in preparation for complete birth.
(A) Placental separation stage
(B) Cervical thinning process
(C) Head realignment movement
(D) Uterine contraction phase
Q412. The Apgar score is used immediately after birth to assess the newborn's condition based on vital physiological criteria.
(A) Newborn status evaluation
(B) Maternal recovery scale
(C) Placental function test
(D) Labor progression tool
Q413. Which factor increases the risk of uterine rupture during labor in a patient attempting vaginal birth after cesarean?
(A) Previous uterine scar
(B) Early labor onset
(C) Reduced maternal age
(D) Mild contraction pattern
Q414. Which intervention is used to artificially stimulate uterine contractions during labor induction or augmentation?
(A) Oxytocin administration
(B) Antibiotic medication use
(C) Insulin infusion therapy
(D) Diuretic drug therapy
Q415. A laboring patient has strong contractions but no progress in fetal descent during the second stage despite adequate pushing efforts. What should be evaluated next to guide clinical management?
(A) Fetal position and alignment
(B) Maternal dietary intake
(C) Contraction frequency pattern
(D) Hydration status level
Q416. A patient receiving epidural analgesia develops hypotension followed by decreased fetal heart rate variability shortly after administration. What is the priority intervention to stabilize maternal and fetal status?

(A) Stop all monitoring immediately
(B) Encourage ambulation
(C) Increase IV fluid infusion
(D) Delay intervention

Q417. A laboring woman receiving oxytocin develops uterine tachysystole with contractions occurring every minute and lasting over 90 seconds. What is the most appropriate action to ensure fetal safety?
(A) Delay response
(B) Encourage ambulation
(C) Discontinue oxytocin infusion
(D) Increase infusion rate

Q418. A newborn presents with jitteriness, weak cry, poor feeding, and laboratory findings indicating low blood glucose levels shortly after birth; what condition is most likely present?
(A) Neonatal hypocalcemia
(B) Neonatal hypoglycemia state
(C) Neonatal infection process
(D) Respiratory distress syndrome

Q419. A laboring patient develops sudden fetal bradycardia immediately after rupture of membranes, and repositioning does not improve the tracing. What is the priority next step in management?
(A) Assess for cord prolapse
(B) Delay further action
(C) Evaluate contraction strength
(D) Monitor maternal diet

Q420. A laboring woman receiving oxytocin suddenly develops severe abdominal pain, vaginal bleeding, cessation of contractions, abnormal fetal heart tracing, and easily palpable fetal parts during active labor. What is the most likely complication requiring immediate surgical intervention?
(A) Uterine rupture emergency
(B) Normal labor progression
(C) Shoulder dystocia event
(D) Cord prolapse condition

Q421. Expulsion occurs when the fetus is completely delivered from the birth canal following coordinated uterine contractions and maternal pushing efforts.
(A) Placental detachment phase
(B) Cervical dilation stage
(C) Uterine relaxation period
(D) Final delivery process

Q422. The placenta is normally delivered during the third stage of labor following separation from the uterine wall after fetal birth.
(A) Contraction initiation phase
(B) Cervical dilation phase
(C) Fetal descent phase
(D) Placental delivery phase

Q423. Which factor increases the likelihood of successful induction of labor in a patient undergoing cervical ripening?
(A) Early fetal movement
(B) Low maternal weight
(C) Reduced contraction strength
(D) Favorable cervical status

Q424. Which intervention is commonly used to manage pain during labor while allowing continuous maternal participation and awareness?
(A) Epidural analgesia method
(B) Complete nerve block
(C) Deep sedation technique
(D) General anesthesia method
Q425. A laboring patient has adequate contractions and full dilation but experiences arrest of descent despite effective pushing. What should be assessed to guide further intervention?
(A) Hydration status level
(B) Frequency of contractions
(C) Fetal position and pelvis
(D) Maternal dietary intake
Q426. A patient receiving epidural analgesia develops hypotension and decreased fetal heart rate variability shortly after administration. What is the priority intervention to improve maternal and fetal status?
(A) Increase IV fluid infusion
(B) Encourage ambulation
(C) Delay intervention
(D) Stop all monitoring
Q427. A laboring woman receiving oxytocin develops contractions every minute with prolonged duration and minimal relaxation between contractions. What is the most appropriate action to ensure fetal safety?
(A) Encourage ambulation
(B) Discontinue oxytocin infusion
(C) Increase infusion rate
(D) Delay response
Q428. A patient undergoing vacuum-assisted delivery requires monitoring for which immediate neonatal complication following birth?
(A) Placental insufficiency
(B) Uterine contraction delay
(C) Umbilical cord compression
(D) Scalp swelling or bruising
Q429. A laboring patient develops sudden fetal bradycardia immediately after rupture of membranes, and repositioning does not improve the condition. What is the priority next step in management?
(A) Delay further action
(B) Assess for cord prolapse
(C) Monitor maternal diet
(D) Evaluate contraction strength
Q430. A laboring woman receiving oxytocin develops sudden severe abdominal pain, vaginal bleeding, cessation of contractions, abnormal fetal heart tracing, and palpable fetal parts during active labor. What is the most likely complication requiring immediate surgical intervention?
(A) Uterine rupture emergency
(B) Cord prolapse condition
(C) Shoulder dystocia event
(D) Normal labor progression
Q431. The third stage of labor involves separation and delivery of the placenta following the birth of the fetus.
(A) Cervical dilation stage

(B) Placental delivery stage
(C) Fetal descent phase
(D) Contraction initiation phase

Q432. Controlled cord traction is a technique used to assist placental delivery while minimizing the risk of uterine inversion.
(A) Cervical dilation method
(B) Assisted placental removal
(C) Contraction stimulation method
(D) Fetal descent technique

Q433. Which condition increases the risk of postpartum hemorrhage during the third stage of labor?
(A) Frequent contractions
(B) Early cervical dilation
(C) Fetal engagement
(D) Uterine atony

Q434. Which intervention is commonly used to promote uterine contraction after delivery of the placenta to prevent hemorrhage?
(A) Diuretic drug therapy
(B) Antibiotic medication use
(C) Oxytocin administration
(D) Insulin infusion therapy

Q435. A patient has delivered the fetus and now shows signs of placental separation, including cord lengthening and a gush of blood. What is the appropriate next step in management?
(A) Assist placental delivery
(B) Assess dietary intake
(C) Begin pushing efforts
(D) Delay intervention

Q436. A patient in the immediate postpartum period develops a soft, boggy uterus with increased vaginal bleeding. What is the priority nursing intervention?
(A) Encourage ambulation
(B) Perform fundal massage
(C) Monitor dietary intake
(D) Delay intervention

Q437. A patient receiving oxytocin postpartum continues to have excessive bleeding despite a firm uterus. What should be evaluated next to determine the cause?
(A) Dietary intake pattern
(B) Maternal hydration level
(C) Genital tract trauma
(D) Frequency of contractions

Q438. A patient who had a vacuum-assisted delivery requires monitoring for which maternal complication immediately after birth?
(A) Umbilical cord compression
(B) Perineal tissue injury
(C) Placental insufficiency
(D) Uterine contraction delay

Q439. A postpartum patient develops sudden heavy vaginal bleeding with a firm uterus and stable vital signs shortly after delivery. What is the priority nursing action to identify the source of bleeding?
(A) Inspect for lacerations
(B) Delay further action

(C) Massage the uterus
(D) Monitor dietary intake

Q440. A postpartum patient suddenly develops severe abdominal pain, signs of shock, and increasing abdominal distension shortly after delivery, with minimal external bleeding. What is the most likely complication requiring immediate intervention?
(A) Normal recovery process
(B) Expected postpartum change
(C) Mild uterine cramping
(D) Internal hemorrhage emergency

Q441. Involution refers to the process by which the uterus returns to its pre-pregnancy size following delivery.
(A) Cervical dilation stage
(B) Placental attachment phase
(C) Fetal descent process
(D) Uterine size reduction

Q442. Lochia is the vaginal discharge that occurs after childbirth as the uterus sheds blood, mucus, and tissue during recovery.
(A) Cervical mucus secretion
(B) Postpartum uterine discharge
(C) Amniotic fluid leakage
(D) Placental blood flow

Q443. Which condition is most commonly associated with delayed postpartum hemorrhage occurring days after delivery?
(A) Strong uterine contractions
(B) Early fetal descent
(C) Retained placental fragments
(D) Normal cervical dilation

Q444. Which intervention is commonly used to stimulate uterine contraction during management of postpartum hemorrhage?
(A) Oxytocin administration
(B) Insulin infusion therapy
(C) Diuretic drug therapy
(D) Antibiotic medication use

Q445. A postpartum patient presents with continued vaginal bleeding and a soft uterus on assessment shortly after delivery. What is the priority nursing action to control bleeding?
(A) Monitor dietary intake
(B) Encourage ambulation
(C) Delay intervention
(D) Perform fundal massage

Q446. A patient continues to bleed heavily postpartum despite a firm uterus and stable vital signs. What should be assessed next to identify the underlying cause?
(A) Dietary intake pattern
(B) Maternal hydration level
(C) Contraction frequency
(D) Genital tract lacerations

Q447. A postpartum patient develops signs of hypovolemia including tachycardia, hypotension, and decreased urine output following delivery. What is the priority intervention to stabilize the patient?
(A) Initiate fluid resuscitation

(B) Delay intervention
(C) Encourage ambulation
(D) Monitor dietary intake

Q448. A patient who underwent operative vaginal delivery reports severe perineal pain and swelling shortly after birth. What complication should be assessed immediately?
(A) Umbilical cord issue
(B) Placental insufficiency
(C) Uterine contraction delay
(D) Hematoma formation

Q449. A postpartum patient develops sudden heavy vaginal bleeding with clots, a firm uterus, and increasing perineal pain within hours after delivery. What is the priority action to identify the cause of bleeding?
(A) Monitor dietary intake
(B) Inspect for hematoma or laceration
(C) Delay intervention
(D) Massage the uterus

Q450. A postpartum patient suddenly develops severe abdominal pain, signs of shock, abdominal distension, and minimal vaginal bleeding shortly after delivery. What is the most likely complication requiring immediate emergency intervention?
(A) Mild uterine cramping
(B) Normal recovery process
(C) Expected postpartum change
(D) Internal hemorrhage emergency

Q451. A laboring patient suddenly reports sharp abdominal pain followed by cessation of contractions and fetal distress; what complication is most likely?
(A) Placental abruption
(B) Placenta previa
(C) Umbilical cord prolapse
(D) Uterine rupture

Q452. A postpartum patient has a soft, boggy uterus and continuous vaginal bleeding; what is the priority intervention?
(A) Encourage ambulation
(B) Perform fundal massage
(C) Initiate breastfeeding
(D) Administer analgesics

Q453. A newborn is placed skin-to-skin immediately after birth; what is the primary purpose of this intervention?
(A) Enhance bonding
(B) Promote early feeding
(C) Maintain body temperature
(D) Prevent infection

Q454. A postpartum patient reports calf pain and swelling; which complication should be suspected?
(A) Urinary tract infection
(B) Deep vein thrombosis
(C) Endometritis
(D) Mastitis

Q455. During labor, recurrent late decelerations are noted on fetal monitoring; what is the priority action?

(A) Position patient supine
(B) Increase oxytocin infusion
(C) Administer oxygen to mother
(D) Encourage pushing

Q456. A newborn has an Apgar score of 5 at one minute; what does this indicate?
(A) Excellent adaptation
(B) Severe distress
(C) No intervention needed
(D) Moderate difficulty

Q457. A postpartum patient develops fever and foul-smelling lochia; what is the likely diagnosis?
(A) Endometritis
(B) Mastitis
(C) Thrombophlebitis
(D) Urinary retention

Q458. A newborn exhibits grunting and nasal flaring shortly after birth; what is the concern?
(A) Respiratory distress
(B) Feeding intolerance
(C) Normal transition
(D) Neurological issue

Q459. A postpartum assessment reveals a firm uterus deviated to the right; what is the likely cause?
(A) Retained placenta
(B) Hemorrhage
(C) Infection
(D) Bladder distention

Q460. During labor, the umbilical cord is visible at the vaginal opening; what is the immediate action?
(A) Continue monitoring
(B) Place patient in knee-chest position
(C) Push the cord back
(D) Prepare for discharge

Q461. A postpartum patient's fundus is firm, midline, and at the level of the umbilicus; how should this finding be interpreted?
(A) Early hemorrhage sign
(B) Normal involution progress
(C) Retained tissue indication
(D) Bladder distention issue

Q462. A newborn is dried immediately after birth; what is the main reason for this action?
(A) Reduce infection
(B) Improve circulation
(C) Enhance bonding
(D) Prevent heat loss

Q463. A patient in labor experiences strong contractions every 2 minutes lasting 90 seconds; what does this indicate?
(A) Active labor progression
(B) Latent phase
(C) False labor
(D) Transition phase

Q464. A postpartum patient reports mild uterine cramping during breastfeeding; what is the cause?
(A) Infection process

(B) Fluid retention
(C) Oxytocin release
(D) Hormonal imbalance

Q465. A laboring patient shows recurrent variable decelerations; what is the most appropriate initial intervention?
(A) Encourage active pushing efforts
(B) Increase IV fluids and reposition patient
(C) Administer sedatives immediately
(D) Prepare for immediate cesarean delivery

Q466. A postpartum patient develops redness and pain in one breast along with fever; what is the likely condition?
(A) Abscess
(B) Mastitis
(C) Engorgement
(D) Hormonal change

Q467. A newborn's Apgar score improves from 6 at one minute to 9 at five minutes; what does this indicate?
(A) Normal adaptation
(B) Severe hypoxia
(C) Immediate emergency
(D) Persistent distress

Q468. A postpartum patient has excessive bleeding despite a firm uterus; what is a possible cause?
(A) Uterine atony
(B) Laceration
(C) Hormonal imbalance
(D) Bladder distention

Q469. A newborn is placed under a radiant warmer; what is the primary purpose of this intervention?
(A) Enhance bonding
(B) Improve feeding
(C) Maintain temperature
(D) Prevent infection

Q470. A patient in labor reports pressure and urge to push; cervical dilation is complete. What is the next step?
(A) Encourage ambulation
(B) Administer analgesia
(C) Delay delivery process
(D) Begin pushing efforts

Q471. A postpartum patient's lochia changes from red to pink by day 4; what does this indicate?
(A) Early infection sign
(B) Delayed involution issue
(C) Normal healing progression
(D) Retained tissue concern

Q472. A newborn exhibits acrocyanosis shortly after birth; what is the interpretation?
(A) Immediate emergency
(B) Circulatory failure
(C) Normal transitional finding
(D) Severe hypoxia sign

Q473. A laboring patient has contractions lasting 60 seconds every 3 minutes with cervical dilation of 6 cm; what stage is this?
(A) Second stage
(B) Latent phase
(C) Transition phase
(D) Active phase
Q474. A postpartum patient experiences chills within the first hour after delivery; what is the likely cause?
(A) Blood loss effect
(B) Fluid imbalance
(C) Hormonal shifts
(D) Infection onset
Q475. A patient in labor develops prolonged decelerations after epidural placement; what is the priority action?
(A) Reposition patient and increase fluids
(B) Encourage pushing immediately
(C) Prepare surgical delivery directly
(D) Administer sedatives promptly
Q476. A postpartum patient reports foul-smelling discharge and uterine tenderness on day 3; what is suspected?
(A) Thrombosis
(B) Normal involution
(C) Endometritis
(D) Mastitis
Q477. A newborn has a heart rate of 90 beats per minute immediately after birth; what does this indicate?
(A) Normal adaptation
(B) Stable condition
(C) Mild compromise
(D) Severe distress
Q478. A postpartum patient's uterus is soft and displaced upward; what action should be taken first?
(A) Begin ambulation
(B) Administer antibiotics
(C) Provide analgesics
(D) Encourage voiding
Q479. A newborn is assessed for reflexes; which reflex involves turning the head when the cheek is touched?
(A) Grasp reflex
(B) Moro reflex
(C) Tonic neck reflex
(D) Rooting reflex
Q480. A laboring patient reports intense rectal pressure and visible crowning is noted; what should the nurse anticipate?
(A) Initiate postpartum care
(B) Transfer to recovery area
(C) Immediate delivery preparation
(D) Delay pushing efforts
Q481. A postpartum patient has lochia alba by the second week; how is this finding interpreted?

(A) Infection development
(B) Early hemorrhage sign
(C) Retained tissue issue
(D) Normal recovery phase

Q482. A newborn's chest circumference is slightly smaller than head circumference; what does this indicate?

(A) Congenital abnormality
(B) Respiratory compromise
(C) Growth restriction sign
(D) Normal physical finding

Q483. A laboring patient has contractions every 5 minutes lasting 40 seconds with minimal cervical change; what phase is this?

(A) Second stage labor
(B) Transition phase stage
(C) Active labor phase
(D) Latent labor phase

Q484. A postpartum patient reports afterpains increasing with multiparity; what explains this occurrence?

(A) Enhanced uterine contractions
(B) Hormonal imbalance
(C) Delayed healing process
(D) Weak uterine tone

Q485. A patient in labor experiences sudden fetal bradycardia after membrane rupture; what is the first action?

(A) Reposition patient immediately
(B) Administer analgesia promptly
(C) Encourage pushing efforts
(D) Prepare for surgery directly

Q486. A postpartum patient complains of painful urination and frequency; what condition is most likely?

(A) Endometritis condition
(B) Deep vein thrombosis
(C) Normal postpartum change
(D) Urinary tract infection

Q487. A newborn demonstrates flexed posture with active movement; what does this indicate?

(A) Respiratory compromise
(B) Poor muscle tone
(C) Severe neurological deficit
(D) Normal neuromuscular function

Q488. A postpartum patient has a temperature of 38.5°C after 24 hours; what should be suspected?

(A) Normal variation
(B) Hormonal fluctuation
(C) Infection presence
(D) Dehydration effect

Q489. A newborn is crying vigorously with pink body color; what does this suggest about adaptation?

(A) Circulatory instability
(B) Respiratory failure
(C) Poor oxygenation

(D) Effective transition

Q490. A laboring patient at full dilation experiences exhaustion and ineffective pushing for over 2 hours; what is the situation?

(A) Early labor phase
(B) Prolonged second stage
(C) Transition phase
(D) Normal labor pattern

Q491. A postpartum patient on day 2 has a firm uterus and moderate lochia rubra without clots; how should this be interpreted?

(A) Delayed involution issue
(B) Early hemorrhage sign
(C) Infection development
(D) Expected postpartum finding

Q492. A newborn maintains a flexed posture with strong cry immediately after birth; what does this indicate about neurological status?

(A) Mild neurological delay
(B) Temporary reflex loss
(C) Normal neurological function
(D) Severe neurological issue

Q493. A laboring patient at 7 cm dilation has contractions every 2-3 minutes lasting 60-70 seconds with increasing intensity; what stage is this?

(A) Second stage labor
(B) Latent labor stage
(C) Active labor stage
(D) Transition phase stage

Q494. A postpartum patient reports mild uterine cramping that intensifies during breastfeeding sessions; what is the physiological cause?

(A) Prolactin hormone release
(B) Progesterone level drop
(C) Estrogen level decrease
(D) Oxytocin hormone action

Q495. A laboring patient develops recurrent late decelerations on fetal monitoring during oxytocin infusion; what should the nurse do first?

(A) Stop oxytocin and reposition patient
(B) Encourage immediate pushing efforts
(C) Prepare for emergency surgery
(D) Administer analgesics quickly

Q496. A postpartum patient on day 3 presents with fever, uterine tenderness, and foul-smelling discharge; what condition is most likely developing?

(A) Uterine infection process
(B) Hormonal imbalance effect
(C) Urinary retention issue
(D) Normal postpartum change

Q497. A newborn's Apgar score is assessed at 1 minute and found to be 8; what does this score indicate about adaptation?

(A) Immediate intervention need
(B) Excellent adaptation status
(C) Moderate distress condition

(D) Severe compromise state

Q498. A postpartum patient's uterus is firm but deviated to the right side above the umbilicus; what is the most appropriate initial nursing action?

(A) Initiate uterine massage

(B) Administer uterotonic drugs

(C) Prepare surgical evaluation

(D) Assist patient to void bladder

Q499. A newborn placed under a radiant warmer maintains stable temperature and normal activity; what does this suggest about thermoregulation?

(A) Effective heat regulation

(B) Increased oxygen demand

(C) Circulatory instability

(D) Poor metabolic function

Q500. A multiparous patient in labor has rapid cervical dilation from 6 cm to full dilation within one hour and begins feeling intense urge to push with rectal pressure; what is the most appropriate interpretation of this situation?

(A) Prolonged labor complication

(B) Rapid labor progression phase

(C) Early latent phase pattern

(D) Ineffective contraction pattern

Answer Key and Explanation (401-500)

Q401. Answer: A
Explanation: Extension is a cardinal movement of labor where the fetal head extends as it passes under the pubic symphysis. This allows the head to be delivered. It follows descent and flexion. Proper alignment supports smooth delivery. Other options describe unrelated processes. ##

Q402. Answer: C
Explanation: External rotation occurs after the head is delivered and realigns with the shoulders. This prepares for delivery of the shoulders. It is one of the final cardinal movements. Proper progression ensures safe birth. Other options are unrelated to this movement. ##

Q403. Answer: A
Explanation: The type of previous uterine incision is critical in VBAC planning. A low transverse incision reduces risk of rupture. Vertical incisions increase complications. Proper assessment ensures safe decision-making. Other factors are less directly related. ##

Q404. Answer: B
Explanation: An intrauterine pressure catheter measures contraction intensity directly. It provides accurate data on uterine activity. It is used when external monitoring is inadequate. Proper placement requires ruptured membranes. Other methods do not measure intensity directly. ##

Q405. Answer: D
Explanation: Failure of descent with adequate contractions suggests possible cephalopelvic disproportion or malposition. Assessing fetal position and pelvic adequacy is essential. This guides decisions such as operative delivery. Early identification prevents complications. Other factors are less directly related. ##

Q406. Answer: D
Explanation: Epidural analgesia can cause vasodilation leading to hypotension. Increasing IV fluids helps restore blood pressure. This improves uteroplacental perfusion and fetal oxygenation. Monitoring is essential. Prompt intervention prevents complications. Other options are inappropriate initially. ##

Q407. Answer: D
Explanation: Tachysystole reduces uterine relaxation and fetal oxygenation. Discontinuing oxytocin helps normalize contraction patterns. Continuous monitoring is essential. Prompt action prevents fetal distress. Other actions may worsen the situation. ##

Q408. Answer: C
Explanation: Blurred vision may indicate hypertensive complications. Postpartum patients remain at risk for preeclampsia. Early recognition is essential for treatment. Patients must be educated on warning signs. Prompt reporting ensures timely care. Monitoring supports patient safety. ##

Q409. Answer: B
Explanation: Persistent fetal bradycardia after membrane rupture suggests cord prolapse. Immediate assessment is critical. Cord compression reduces fetal oxygenation. Rapid intervention improves outcomes. Other actions are secondary. Prompt recognition is essential. ##

Q410. Answer: D
Explanation: Severe pain, bleeding, and abnormal fetal tracing indicate uterine rupture. Palpable fetal parts confirm uterine wall disruption. This is a life-threatening emergency. Immediate surgical intervention is required. Delay increases risk of maternal and fetal mortality. Early recognition improves outcomes significantly. ##

Q411. Answer: C
Explanation: Restitution is the movement where the fetal head rotates after delivery to align with the shoulders. It follows extension and prepares for shoulder delivery. This movement reflects internal

rotation of the shoulders. Proper sequence ensures smooth birth. Other options describe unrelated processes. ##

Q412. Answer: A

Explanation: The Apgar score evaluates the newborn's condition at 1 and 5 minutes after birth. It includes heart rate, respiration, muscle tone, reflex response, and color. This helps determine the need for immediate care. It is a rapid and essential assessment tool. Other options are incorrect uses. ##

Q413. Answer: A

Explanation: A previous uterine scar weakens the uterine wall and increases rupture risk. This is especially relevant during VBAC. Careful monitoring is required during labor. Other factors do not significantly increase rupture risk. Proper patient selection improves safety. ##

Q414. Answer: A

Explanation: Oxytocin is used to induce or augment labor by stimulating uterine contractions. It increases contraction frequency and strength. Careful monitoring is essential to avoid complications. It is widely used in obstetric care. Other medications do not have this effect. ##

Q415. Answer: A

Explanation: Lack of descent despite strong contractions suggests malposition or obstruction. Assessing fetal position helps identify alignment issues. This guides repositioning or assisted delivery. Other factors are less directly related. Early evaluation improves outcomes. ##

Q416. Answer: C

Explanation: Epidural analgesia can cause vasodilation leading to hypotension. Increasing IV fluids helps restore blood pressure. This improves uteroplacental perfusion and fetal oxygenation. Continuous monitoring is essential. Prompt action prevents complications. Other options are not appropriate initially. ##

Q417. Answer: C

Explanation: Tachysystole reduces uterine relaxation time and fetal oxygenation. Discontinuing oxytocin helps restore normal contraction patterns. Continuous monitoring is essential. Prompt intervention prevents fetal distress. Other actions may worsen the situation. ##

Q418. Answer: B

Explanation: Hypoglycemia affects neurological stability in newborns. Symptoms include jitteriness and poor feeding. A weak cry may also be present. Early detection is essential to prevent complications. Treatment includes feeding or glucose administration. Monitoring ensures stabilization of glucose levels. ##

Q419. Answer: A

Explanation: Persistent fetal bradycardia after membrane rupture suggests cord prolapse. Immediate assessment is critical. Cord compression compromises fetal oxygenation. Rapid intervention improves outcomes. Other actions are secondary. Prompt recognition is essential in emergencies. ##

Q420. Answer: A

Explanation: Severe pain, bleeding, and abnormal fetal tracing indicate uterine rupture. Palpable fetal parts confirm uterine wall disruption. This is a life-threatening emergency. Immediate surgical intervention is required. Delay increases risk of maternal and fetal mortality. Early recognition improves outcomes significantly. ##

Q421. Answer: D

Explanation: Expulsion refers to the complete delivery of the fetus from the birth canal. It occurs at the end of the second stage of labor. Coordinated contractions and maternal pushing facilitate this process. It marks the transition to the third stage. Other options describe different phases. ##

Q422. Answer: D

Explanation: The third stage of labor involves delivery of the placenta. It begins after the fetus is born. Uterine contractions help detach and expel the placenta. Proper management reduces risk of hemorrhage. Other options refer to earlier labor processes. ##

Q423. Answer: D

Explanation: A favorable cervix increases the success of labor induction. This includes softening, dilation, and effacement. It is often assessed using scoring systems. Better cervical readiness leads to effective contractions. Other factors are less predictive. ##

Q424. Answer: A

Explanation: Epidural analgesia provides effective pain relief while maintaining consciousness. It allows the patient to participate in labor. It is widely used in obstetric care. Monitoring is required for side effects. Other methods reduce awareness or are not continuous. ##

Q425. Answer: C

Explanation: Arrest of descent suggests possible malposition or cephalopelvic disproportion. Assessing fetal position and pelvic adequacy is essential. This guides decisions such as assisted delivery or cesarean section. Early evaluation prevents complications. Other factors are less directly related. ##

Q426. Answer: A

Explanation: Epidural anesthesia can cause vasodilation leading to hypotension. Increasing IV fluids helps restore blood pressure. This improves uteroplacental perfusion and fetal oxygenation. Continuous monitoring is essential. Prompt action prevents complications. Other options are inappropriate initially. ##

Q427. Answer: B

Explanation: Excessive contractions reduce uterine relaxation time and fetal oxygenation. Discontinuing oxytocin helps normalize contraction patterns. Continuous monitoring is essential. Prompt intervention prevents fetal distress. Other actions may worsen the condition. ##

Q428. Answer: D

Explanation: Vacuum extraction can cause scalp swelling or bruising in the newborn. These findings are usually temporary but require monitoring. Proper technique reduces risk. Immediate newborn assessment is essential. Other options are not directly related. ##

Q429. Answer: B

Explanation: Persistent fetal bradycardia after membrane rupture suggests cord prolapse. Immediate assessment is critical. Cord compression compromises fetal oxygenation. Rapid intervention improves outcomes. Other actions are secondary. Prompt recognition is essential in emergencies. ##

Q430. Answer: A

Explanation: Severe abdominal pain, bleeding, and abnormal fetal tracing indicate uterine rupture. Palpable fetal parts confirm uterine wall disruption. This is a life-threatening emergency. Immediate surgical intervention is required. Delay increases risk of maternal and fetal mortality. Early recognition improves outcomes significantly. ##

Q431. Answer: B

Explanation: The third stage begins after fetal delivery and ends with placental expulsion. Uterine contractions help detach the placenta from the uterine wall. Proper management reduces risk of hemorrhage. Monitoring for complete placental delivery is essential. Other options refer to earlier labor processes. ##

Q432. Answer: B

Explanation: Controlled cord traction gently assists in delivering the placenta. It is performed while supporting the uterus. This reduces risk of uterine inversion. Proper technique improves safety during the third stage. Other options describe unrelated processes. ##

Q433. Answer: D

Explanation: Uterine atony is the most common cause of postpartum hemorrhage. The uterus fails to contract effectively after delivery. This leads to excessive bleeding. Prompt recognition and treatment are essential. Other factors are less directly associated. ##

Q434. Answer: C

Explanation: Oxytocin is administered after delivery to stimulate uterine contractions. This helps compress blood vessels and reduce bleeding. It is a standard preventive measure. Monitoring ensures effectiveness. Other medications do not have this effect. ##

Q435. Answer: A

Explanation: Signs of placental separation indicate readiness for delivery. Controlled assistance helps expel the placenta safely. This prevents retained placenta and bleeding. Monitoring uterine tone is essential. Other actions are not appropriate at this stage. ##

Q436. Answer: B

Explanation: A boggy uterus indicates uterine atony, leading to hemorrhage. Fundal massage stimulates contraction and reduces bleeding. Prompt action is essential. Additional medications may be required. Other actions are secondary. Early intervention prevents complications. ##

Q437. Answer: C

Explanation: Excessive bleeding with a firm uterus suggests trauma rather than atony. Lacerations or hematomas should be assessed. Identifying the source guides treatment. Prompt intervention prevents further blood loss. Other factors are less directly related. ##

Q438. Answer: B

Explanation: Vacuum-assisted delivery can cause perineal or vaginal trauma. Monitoring for bleeding and tissue injury is essential. Proper technique reduces risk. Early detection allows prompt management. Other complications are less directly related. ##

Q439. Answer: A

Explanation: Heavy bleeding with a firm uterus suggests lacerations. Inspecting the genital tract helps identify the source. Uterine massage is not effective in this case. Prompt identification allows appropriate repair. Other actions are secondary. Early intervention prevents complications. ##

Q440. Answer: D

Explanation: Severe pain, shock, and abdominal distension suggest internal hemorrhage. Blood may accumulate internally with minimal external signs. This is a life-threatening condition. Immediate intervention is required. Delay increases risk of maternal mortality. Early recognition is critical. ##

Q441. Answer: D

Explanation: Involution is the gradual shrinking of the uterus after childbirth. It begins immediately after delivery of the placenta. Effective uterine contractions support this process. It helps prevent excessive bleeding. Other options describe unrelated labor processes. ##

Q442. Answer: B

Explanation: Lochia is the normal postpartum discharge consisting of blood and uterine tissue. It changes in color and amount over time. This reflects uterine healing. Monitoring helps identify abnormal bleeding. Other options describe unrelated fluids. ##

Q443. Answer: C

Explanation: Retained placental fragments can prevent proper uterine contraction. This leads to delayed postpartum hemorrhage. Symptoms may appear days after delivery. Prompt diagnosis and treatment are required. Other options are not associated with delayed bleeding. ##

Q444. Answer: A

Explanation: Oxytocin stimulates uterine contractions and helps control bleeding. It is the first-line treatment for postpartum hemorrhage. It promotes uterine tone. Monitoring ensures effectiveness. Other medications do not have this action. ##

Q445. Answer: D

Explanation: A soft uterus indicates uterine atony, the leading cause of postpartum hemorrhage. Fundal massage stimulates contraction and reduces bleeding. Immediate action is essential. Additional medications may be required. Other actions are secondary. Early intervention prevents complications. ##

Q446. Answer: D

Explanation: Heavy bleeding with a firm uterus suggests trauma such as lacerations. Inspection of the genital tract is essential. Identifying the source guides treatment. Prompt intervention prevents further blood loss. Other factors are less relevant. Early detection is critical. ##

Q447. Answer: A

Explanation: Signs of hypovolemia indicate significant blood loss. Fluid resuscitation restores circulating volume. This stabilizes blood pressure and organ perfusion. Rapid intervention is essential. Additional treatment may be required. Other options are not appropriate initially. ##

Q448. Answer: D

Explanation: Severe pain and swelling suggest hematoma formation. This can occur after operative delivery. It may lead to concealed bleeding. Prompt assessment is required. Early management prevents complications. Other options are less directly related. ##

Q449. Answer: B

Explanation: Heavy bleeding with a firm uterus suggests trauma or hematoma. Inspection helps identify the source. Uterine massage is not effective in this case. Prompt diagnosis allows appropriate treatment. Other actions are secondary. Early intervention prevents complications. ##

Q450. Answer: D

Explanation: Severe pain, shock, and distension suggest internal hemorrhage. Blood may accumulate internally with little external bleeding. This is a life-threatening condition. Immediate intervention is required. Delay increases mortality risk. Early recognition is critical for survival. ##

Q451. Answer: D

Explanation: Sudden intense abdominal pain combined with loss of contractions is a classic presentation of uterine rupture. This condition results in disruption of the uterine wall, leading to fetal compromise. Fetal distress occurs due to impaired oxygen delivery after rupture. Immediate surgical intervention is required to prevent maternal and fetal mortality. The clinical picture also includes abnormal abdominal contour and possible loss of fetal station. Prompt recognition is critical for survival outcomes. ##

Q452. Answer: B

Explanation: A boggy uterus indicates uterine atony, which is the most common cause of postpartum hemorrhage. Fundal massage stimulates uterine contraction and helps control bleeding. Immediate action is necessary to prevent excessive blood loss and shock. This intervention is non-invasive and can quickly restore uterine tone. Continuous assessment is required to ensure effectiveness. Additional medications may be needed if the response is inadequate. ##

Q453. Answer: C

Explanation: Skin-to-skin contact helps stabilize the newborn's temperature by reducing heat loss. Newborns are highly susceptible to hypothermia due to immature thermoregulation. Maintaining warmth supports metabolic stability and oxygen consumption. This intervention also indirectly supports breastfeeding initiation. It is a simple yet highly effective practice in immediate newborn care. Consistent thermal regulation reduces neonatal complications. ##

Q454. Answer: B

Explanation: Calf pain and swelling in the postpartum period are hallmark signs of deep vein thrombosis. Hypercoagulability during pregnancy increases the risk of clot formation. Early recognition is important to prevent progression to pulmonary embolism. Assessment includes checking for warmth, redness, and tenderness. Immobilization and anticoagulation therapy are typically required. Prompt medical evaluation is essential for patient safety. ##

Q455. Answer: C

Explanation: Late decelerations indicate uteroplacental insufficiency and fetal hypoxia. Administering oxygen improves maternal oxygenation and fetal supply. Immediate interventions aim to enhance placental perfusion. Continuous monitoring is necessary to evaluate response. Additional steps may include repositioning and stopping uterotonic agents. Timely intervention prevents worsening fetal distress. ##

Q456. Answer: D

Explanation: An Apgar score of 5 reflects moderate difficulty in adapting to extrauterine life. This score suggests the need for some supportive interventions. Assessment includes heart rate, respiration, muscle tone, reflex response, and color. Continuous reassessment at five minutes is essential. Improvement indicates successful adaptation. Early intervention helps prevent complications. ##

Q457. Answer: A

Explanation: Fever with foul-smelling lochia is characteristic of endometritis. This infection affects the uterine lining after delivery. Risk factors include prolonged labor and retained placental fragments. Early treatment with antibiotics is necessary to prevent spread. Monitoring vital signs and uterine tenderness aids diagnosis. Prompt care improves recovery outcomes. ##

Q458. Answer: A

Explanation: Grunting and nasal flaring are signs of respiratory distress in a newborn. These symptoms indicate increased effort to maintain adequate oxygenation. Early detection allows for prompt respiratory support. Conditions like transient tachypnea or respiratory distress syndrome may be present. Continuous monitoring is essential for stabilization. Immediate care reduces risk of complications. ##

Q459. Answer: D

Explanation: A firm but displaced uterus is commonly due to a full bladder. Bladder distention pushes the uterus to one side, affecting its position. This can interfere with uterine contraction and increase bleeding risk. Encouraging voiding helps return the uterus to midline. Assessment of urinary status is essential postpartum. Early correction prevents complications. ##

Q460. Answer: B

Explanation: A visible umbilical cord indicates cord prolapse, a medical emergency. Knee-chest positioning reduces pressure on the cord and improves blood flow. Maintaining oxygen supply to the fetus is critical. Immediate preparation for emergency delivery is required. Continuous fetal monitoring is essential. Rapid intervention improves fetal outcomes. ##

Q461. Answer: B

Explanation: A firm, midline uterus at the umbilicus is an expected finding shortly after delivery. This indicates effective uterine contraction and normal involution. Proper uterine tone helps prevent excessive bleeding. Consistent assessment ensures the uterus remains firm over time. Any deviation from this pattern may require intervention. This finding reflects a stable postpartum condition. ##

Q462. Answer: D

Explanation: Drying the newborn removes amniotic fluid that contributes to evaporative heat loss. Newborns have limited ability to regulate temperature. Preventing hypothermia is essential for metabolic stability. Maintaining warmth reduces oxygen consumption. This simple intervention plays a critical role in early neonatal care. Consistent thermal management improves outcomes. ##

Q463. Answer: D

Explanation: Frequent, intense contractions occurring every two minutes are characteristic of the transition phase. This stage represents the final part of the first stage of labor. Cervical dilation is nearly complete during this time. The intensity often leads to increased discomfort and emotional changes. Close monitoring is essential for maternal and fetal well-being. This phase signals imminent delivery. ##

Q464. Answer: C

Explanation: Breastfeeding stimulates oxytocin release, which causes uterine contractions. These contractions help the uterus return to its pre-pregnancy size. This process also reduces the risk of postpartum hemorrhage. Mild cramping is a common and expected response. The sensation typically decreases over time. It reflects a normal physiological mechanism aiding recovery. ##

Q465. Answer: B

Explanation: Variable decelerations are commonly caused by umbilical cord compression. Repositioning the patient can relieve pressure on the cord. Increasing IV fluids may improve placental perfusion. Continuous monitoring is necessary to assess response. Early interventions aim to stabilize fetal heart patterns. Prompt correction reduces risk of fetal compromise. ##

Q466. Answer: B

Explanation: Breast redness, pain, and fever are classic signs of mastitis. This condition results from infection of breast tissue. It often occurs due to milk stasis or bacterial entry. Early treatment includes antibiotics and continued breastfeeding. Proper hygiene and complete emptying of the breast help prevent recurrence. Prompt management reduces complications. ##

Q467. Answer: A

Explanation: Improvement in Apgar score indicates successful adaptation to extrauterine life. The increase reflects better respiratory effort, heart rate, and muscle tone. Monitoring over time helps evaluate newborn stability. A higher score at five minutes suggests effective transition. Minimal intervention is typically required after improvement. This trend is a positive clinical sign. ##

Q468. Answer: B

Explanation: Excessive bleeding with a firm uterus often indicates trauma such as lacerations. Tears in the cervix, vagina, or perineum can cause continuous bleeding. Assessment should include inspection for visible injury. Prompt repair is necessary to control blood loss. This differs from atony, where the uterus is soft. Early identification prevents complications. ##

Q469. Answer: C

Explanation: A radiant warmer helps maintain the newborn's body temperature. Newborns are prone to rapid heat loss due to large surface area. Controlled warmth prevents cold stress and metabolic complications. It allows for easy access during assessment and care. Continuous monitoring ensures thermal stability. This intervention supports safe neonatal transition. ##

Q470. Answer: D

Explanation: Full cervical dilation with urge to push indicates the second stage of labor. Active pushing helps facilitate fetal descent and delivery. Proper guidance ensures effective efforts and reduces fatigue. Continuous monitoring of fetal status is essential. This stage progresses toward birth. Timely action supports safe delivery outcomes. ##

Q471. Answer: C

Explanation: Lochia typically transitions from red to pink within a few days after delivery. This change reflects normal healing and uterine recovery. The progression indicates decreasing blood content and increasing serous fluid. Continuous monitoring ensures the pattern remains appropriate. Any reversal or abnormal odor would require evaluation. This finding supports normal postpartum recovery. ##

Q472. Answer: C

Explanation: Acrocyanosis refers to bluish discoloration of the hands and feet in newborns. It is a common and temporary condition during early adaptation. Peripheral circulation takes time to stabilize after birth. Central color remains pink, which is reassuring. Continuous observation ensures no progression to central cyanosis. This finding is generally benign and self-limiting. ##

Q473. Answer: D

Explanation: Contractions every three minutes with moderate duration indicate active labor. Cervical dilation of 6 cm supports this stage classification. This phase involves steady progression toward full dilation. Monitoring contraction pattern helps assess labor efficiency. Pain intensity often increases during this time. Proper support is essential for maternal comfort and progress. ##

Q474. Answer: C

Explanation: Postpartum chills are commonly due to rapid hormonal changes after delivery. These shifts affect the body's temperature regulation temporarily. The phenomenon is usually short-lived and resolves spontaneously. Vital signs should still be monitored to rule out complications. No specific treatment is typically required. This response is considered a normal physiological adjustment. ##

Q475. Answer: A

Explanation: Epidural anesthesia can lead to hypotension, reducing placental perfusion. Repositioning improves circulation and venous return. Increasing IV fluids helps stabilize blood pressure. Continuous monitoring evaluates fetal response to intervention. Early correction can restore normal heart rate patterns. Prompt action minimizes fetal compromise risk. ##

Q476. Answer: C

Explanation: Foul-smelling discharge with uterine tenderness suggests infection of the uterine lining. This condition commonly occurs within the first few days postpartum. Risk factors include prolonged labor and invasive procedures. Early antibiotic therapy is essential to control infection. Monitoring for fever and systemic symptoms is necessary. Prompt treatment prevents further complications. ##

Q477. Answer: C

Explanation: A heart rate below 100 beats per minute indicates some level of compromise. Immediate assessment and supportive measures are required. Stimulation or ventilation may be necessary to improve status. Continuous reassessment ensures improvement. Early intervention helps stabilize the newborn. This finding requires prompt attention but is often reversible. ##

Q478. Answer: D

Explanation: A soft and displaced uterus often results from bladder distention. Encouraging voiding relieves pressure and allows the uterus to contract properly. Restoring uterine tone reduces bleeding risk. Assessment should follow to confirm improvement. Early intervention prevents complications. Bladder management is essential in postpartum care. ##

Q479. Answer: D

Explanation: The rooting reflex helps the newborn locate a food source. Touching the cheek triggers head turning toward the stimulus. This reflex supports successful feeding behavior. It is present at birth and fades over time. Assessment confirms neurological integrity. Normal presence indicates appropriate development. ##

Q480. Answer: C

Explanation: Crowning indicates the fetal head is visible at the vaginal opening. This signals that birth is imminent. Preparation for delivery ensures safety for both mother and newborn. Necessary equipment and personnel should be ready. Continuous support is essential during this stage. Rapid progression requires prompt readiness. ##

Q481. Answer: D

Explanation: Lochia alba represents the final stage of postpartum discharge. It typically appears as a whitish or yellowish fluid after the initial stages. This indicates that the uterus is nearing complete healing. The reduction in blood content reflects proper involution. Continued monitoring ensures no abnormal changes occur. This finding supports a normal recovery process. ##

Q482. Answer: D

Explanation: In newborns, the head circumference is normally larger than the chest circumference. This is due to brain growth and developmental proportions. The difference is usually about 2 to 3 centimeters. This finding is expected and does not indicate pathology. Regular measurements help track growth trends. It reflects normal neonatal anatomy. ##

Q483. Answer: D

Explanation: Contractions that are mild, spaced apart, and with slow cervical change indicate the latent phase. This early stage of labor can last several hours. Cervical dilation progresses gradually during this time. Comfort measures and support are important. Monitoring ensures progression continues appropriately. This phase precedes more active labor. ##

Q484. Answer: A

Explanation: Afterpains are more pronounced in multiparous patients due to stronger uterine contractions. The uterus must work harder to return to its pre-pregnancy size. Repeated stretching from prior pregnancies contributes to this effect. These contractions help reduce bleeding. The discomfort is usually temporary and manageable. This response reflects normal physiology. ##

Q485. Answer: A

Explanation: Sudden fetal bradycardia after membrane rupture may indicate cord compression or prolapse. Repositioning helps relieve pressure and improve blood flow. Immediate intervention is essential to restore fetal oxygenation. Continuous monitoring evaluates response to action. Additional steps may be needed if no improvement occurs. Early management reduces fetal risk. ##

Q486. Answer: D

Explanation: Painful urination and increased frequency are common signs of urinary tract infection. Postpartum patients are at higher risk due to catheter use or trauma. Early diagnosis helps prevent complications. Treatment typically involves antibiotics and hydration. Monitoring symptoms ensures resolution. Prompt care improves patient comfort and outcomes. ##

Q487. Answer: D

Explanation: A flexed posture with active movement indicates good muscle tone in a newborn. This is a sign of normal neuromuscular development. Healthy newborns maintain flexion due to intrauterine positioning. Active movement reflects intact neurological function. Assessment of tone is part of routine evaluation. This finding is reassuring for overall health. ##

Q488. Answer: C

Explanation: A temperature above 38°C after the first 24 hours postpartum suggests infection. Common sources include uterine or urinary infections. Early identification is important for timely treatment. Monitoring additional symptoms helps determine the cause. Antibiotic therapy may be required. Prompt management prevents progression. ##

Q489. Answer: D

Explanation: Vigorous crying and pink coloration indicate effective oxygenation. These signs reflect successful adaptation to extrauterine life. Adequate respiratory effort ensures proper gas exchange. Circulatory adjustments are functioning well. Continued observation confirms stability. This is a positive indicator of newborn health. ##

Q490. Answer: B

Explanation: Ineffective pushing for an extended period indicates prolonged second stage of labor. This can increase risk for both mother and fetus. Monitoring for signs of distress is essential. Interventions may be required to assist delivery. Fatigue contributes to decreased effectiveness of pushing. Timely management supports safe outcomes. ##

Q491. Answer: D

Explanation: A firm uterus with moderate lochia rubra during the first few days postpartum is considered normal. This indicates that the uterus is contracting effectively and shedding its lining appropriately. The absence of large clots further supports stable recovery. Continuous monitoring ensures that bleeding does not increase unexpectedly. Normal progression involves gradual reduction in flow over time. This finding reflects healthy postpartum adaptation. ##

Q492. Answer: C

Explanation: A strong cry combined with flexed posture reflects intact neurological function in a newborn. These signs indicate appropriate muscle tone and central nervous system activity. Normal reflexes and movement patterns support this assessment. Continuous evaluation ensures sustained adaptation. This presentation is expected in healthy newborns. It confirms proper early neurological development. ##

Q493. Answer: C

Explanation: Cervical dilation of 7 cm with strong, frequent contractions indicates active labor. This phase is characterized by rapid cervical change and increased discomfort. The contraction pattern supports effective progression toward full dilation. Monitoring ensures both maternal and fetal well-being. Support measures are important to manage pain and fatigue. This stage precedes the transition phase. ##

Q494. Answer: D

Explanation: Breastfeeding stimulates oxytocin release, which causes uterine contractions. These contractions help reduce uterine size and minimize bleeding. Increased intensity during feeding is expected due to repeated hormone release. This mechanism supports efficient postpartum recovery. The discomfort usually decreases over time. It reflects a normal and beneficial physiological process. ##

Q495. Answer: A

Explanation: Late decelerations indicate reduced oxygen supply to the fetus. Stopping oxytocin decreases uterine stimulation and improves blood flow. Repositioning enhances placental perfusion and oxygen delivery. Continuous monitoring is required to assess improvement. Early intervention can reverse fetal distress. Prompt action is critical to prevent further complications. ##

Q496. Answer: A

Explanation: Fever with uterine tenderness and foul discharge strongly suggests uterine infection. This condition typically occurs within a few days after delivery. Risk factors include prolonged labor and invasive procedures. Early treatment with antibiotics is essential to control infection. Monitoring systemic symptoms ensures timely response. Prompt care prevents serious complications. ##

Q497. Answer: B

Explanation: An Apgar score of 8 indicates that the newborn is adapting well to extrauterine life. Most physiological functions such as heart rate and respiration are stable. Minor adjustments may still be occurring but do not require major intervention. Continued monitoring ensures stability. Reassessment at five minutes confirms progress. This score reflects a healthy transition. ##

Q498. Answer: D

Explanation: A firm uterus that is displaced from the midline often indicates bladder distention. Assisting the patient to void relieves pressure and allows the uterus to return to its normal position. Proper alignment supports effective uterine contraction. This helps reduce the risk of excessive bleeding. Follow-up assessment ensures correction. Early intervention promotes optimal recovery. ##

Q499. Answer: A

Explanation: Stable temperature under a radiant warmer indicates effective thermoregulation. The newborn is maintaining appropriate body heat with external support. This prevents cold stress and metabolic imbalance. Adequate temperature control supports oxygen efficiency. Continuous monitoring ensures ongoing stability. This finding reflects successful neonatal adaptation. ##

Q500. Answer: B

Explanation: Rapid cervical dilation with strong urge to push indicates accelerated labor progression. Multiparous patients often experience faster labor due to prior uterine stretching. Intense rectal pressure suggests fetal descent into the birth canal. Immediate preparation for delivery is necessary. Continuous monitoring ensures safety for both mother and fetus. This situation reflects efficient but rapid labor progression. ## Question (501-600)

Question (501-600)

Q501. A postpartum patient's fundus is firm and located one fingerbreadth below the umbilicus on day 1; what does this indicate?
(A) Infection development
(B) Normal uterine involution
(C) Retained placenta sign
(D) Early hemorrhage risk
Q502. A newborn's skin appears slightly bluish on hands and feet but pink centrally; what is this finding called?
(A) Circulatory failure state
(B) Severe hypoxia sign
(C) Central cyanosis state
(D) Peripheral acrocyanosis finding
Q503. A patient at 5 cm dilation has contractions every 4 minutes lasting 50 seconds and reports increasing discomfort; how should this labor pattern be interpreted?
(A) Early latent phase
(B) Active labor phase
(C) Second stage labor
(D) Transition stage onset
Q504. A postpartum patient reports increased vaginal bleeding after ambulating, but the uterus remains firm on assessment; what is the most likely explanation?
(A) Uterine atony presence
(B) Normal pooled blood release
(C) Infection development process
(D) Coagulation disorder onset
Q505. A laboring patient receiving oxytocin develops contractions every 1 minute lasting 100 seconds with minimal resting tone; what is the priority nursing action?
(A) Continue monitoring contractions
(B) Discontinue oxytocin infusion immediately
(C) Encourage deep breathing exercises
(D) Assist patient with ambulation
Q506. A postpartum patient on day 4 develops localized breast pain, redness, and fever; what underlying process is occurring?
(A) Normal milk production
(B) Hormonal fluctuation
(C) Infectious inflammation
(D) Circulatory congestion
Q507. A newborn exhibits a strong suck reflex and coordinated swallowing during feeding; what does this indicate?
(A) Gastrointestinal disorder
(B) Respiratory compromise
(C) Normal neurological coordination
(D) Poor feeding ability
Q508. A postpartum patient has a temperature of 38.2°C within the first 12 hours after delivery but no other symptoms; how should this be interpreted?
(A) Normal transient response
(B) Likely infection onset

(C) Severe complication sign
(D) Immediate emergency

Q509. A newborn is placed skin-to-skin with the mother immediately after birth and maintains stable vital signs; what is the primary benefit of this practice?
(A) Eliminates need for monitoring
(B) Accelerates reflex development
(C) Prevents immediate infection
(D) Enhances thermoregulation stability

Q510. A multiparous patient arrives in labor reporting contractions every 2 minutes for the past hour, strong urge to push, and increasing rectal pressure; on examination, the cervix is fully dilated and fetal head is at +2 station. What is the most appropriate nursing action at this time?
(A) Delay pushing until provider arrives
(B) Encourage ambulation for comfort
(C) Prepare immediately for delivery
(D) Transfer patient to recovery unit

Q511. A postpartum patient has a firm uterus located at the umbilicus immediately after delivery; how is this finding interpreted?
(A) Early hemorrhage sign
(B) Infection indication
(C) Normal postpartum status
(D) Delayed involution

Q512. A newborn demonstrates rooting when the cheek is stroked; what does this reflex support?
(A) Circulatory stability
(B) Temperature regulation
(C) Respiratory adaptation
(D) Feeding behavior initiation

Q513. A patient at 6 cm dilation reports stronger contractions every 3 minutes lasting 60 seconds and increasing discomfort; how should this labor stage be interpreted?
(A) Latent phase stage
(B) Second stage labor
(C) Active labor phase
(D) Transition phase stage

Q514. A postpartum patient notices a sudden gush of dark blood upon standing, but the uterus remains firm on palpation; what is the likely explanation?
(A) Normal pooled blood release
(B) Uterine atony
(C) Coagulation disorder
(D) Infection process

Q515. A laboring patient receiving oxytocin develops a contraction pattern with minimal relaxation between contractions and signs of fetal distress; what should be done first?
(A) Encourage pushing efforts
(B) Administer analgesia promptly
(C) Continue infusion as ordered
(D) Stop oxytocin and reposition

Q516. A postpartum patient on day 5 reports breast engorgement without fever or redness; what is the underlying cause of this condition?
(A) Circulatory obstruction
(B) Milk accumulation process

(C) Infection development
(D) Hormonal deficiency
Q517. A newborn exhibits spontaneous movement, strong cry, and good muscle tone shortly after birth; what does this indicate?
(A) Effective neonatal transition
(B) Poor adaptation status
(C) Severe neurological deficit
(D) Respiratory compromise
Q518. A postpartum patient presents with persistent fever, uterine tenderness, and malaise three days after delivery; how should this condition be interpreted?
(A) Normal postpartum response
(B) Hormonal adjustment phase
(C) Uterine infection presence
(D) Mild dehydration state
Q519. A newborn is placed under a radiant warmer and maintains stable oxygen saturation and temperature; what does this indicate about neonatal adaptation?
(A) Stable physiological adjustment
(B) Ineffective thermoregulation
(C) Increased metabolic stress
(D) Circulatory compromise
Q520. A multiparous patient arrives at the labor unit reporting intense contractions every 2 minutes for the past hour, inability to talk during contractions, and a strong urge to push; examination reveals full cervical dilation and the fetal head at +3 station. What is the most appropriate immediate nursing action?
(A) Delay pushing until reassessment
(B) Encourage rest and breathing
(C) Transfer patient for observation
(D) Prepare for immediate delivery
Q521. A postpartum patient has a firm uterus and scant lochia serosa on day 5; what does this indicate?
(A) Retained tissue issue
(B) Early hemorrhage risk
(C) Normal healing progress
(D) Infection development
Q522. A newborn exhibits a Moro reflex when startled; what does this reflex indicate?
(A) Feeding difficulty
(B) Respiratory distress sign
(C) Circulatory instability
(D) Neurological integrity present
Q523. A laboring patient is at 8 cm dilation with contractions every 2 minutes lasting 70 seconds and increasing intensity; how should this stage be interpreted?
(A) Second stage labor
(B) Transition phase stage
(C) Active labor phase
(D) Latent phase stage
Q524. A postpartum patient reports increased bleeding after breastfeeding, but the uterus remains firm and midline; what explains this finding?
(A) Normal uterine response

(B) Infection progression
(C) Retained placenta
(D) Coagulation disorder

Q525. A patient in labor receiving oxytocin develops contractions every minute lasting over 90 seconds with signs of fetal distress; what is the priority action?
(A) Encourage breathing techniques
(B) Prepare discharge planning
(C) Stop oxytocin infusion immediately
(D) Continue monitoring closely

Q526. A postpartum patient on day 4 develops localized breast tenderness without fever and firm areas are palpated; what condition is most likely present?
(A) Vascular obstruction
(B) Early engorgement stage
(C) Hormonal imbalance
(D) Infectious mastitis

Q527. A newborn demonstrates coordinated suck, swallow, and breathing during feeding sessions; what does this indicate?
(A) Normal feeding ability
(B) Respiratory compromise
(C) Gastrointestinal issue
(D) Neurological deficit

Q528. A postpartum patient develops a fever of 38.3°C on day 3 with uterine tenderness and fatigue; how should this condition be interpreted?
(A) Infection presence
(B) Dehydration effect
(C) Normal postpartum change
(D) Hormonal fluctuation

Q529. A newborn maintains stable temperature, heart rate, and respiratory effort within the first hour after birth; what does this suggest about transition?
(A) Delayed adjustment
(B) Successful adaptation
(C) Circulatory failure
(D) Respiratory distress

Q530. A multiparous patient arrives at the unit reporting contractions every 2 minutes for 90 minutes, inability to speak during contractions, increasing rectal pressure, and an urge to bear down; on examination, cervix is fully dilated and fetal head is at +3 station with visible crowning. What is the most appropriate immediate nursing action?
(A) Encourage rest and breathing
(B) Prepare for immediate delivery
(C) Delay pushing until provider arrives
(D) Transfer patient to another unit

Q531. A postpartum patient's uterus is firm and located 2 cm below the umbilicus on day 2; what does this finding indicate?
(A) Normal involution process
(B) Delayed uterine recovery
(C) Early hemorrhage sign
(D) Retained tissue concern

Q532. A newborn displays a palmar grasp reflex when an object is placed in the hand; what does this indicate?
(A) Circulatory issue
(B) Feeding difficulty
(C) Neurological impairment
(D) Normal reflex activity
Q533. A patient in labor at 4 cm dilation reports contractions every 5 minutes lasting 45 seconds with mild discomfort; how should this stage be interpreted?
(A) Transition phase labor
(B) Second stage labor
(C) Active phase labor
(D) Latent phase labor
Q534. A postpartum patient notices increased bleeding when moving from lying to standing, but the uterus remains firm and midline on assessment; what is the most likely explanation?
(A) Infection development
(B) Normal pooled blood release
(C) Coagulation disorder
(D) Uterine atony condition
Q535. A laboring patient receiving oxytocin develops contractions every minute lasting 100 seconds with minimal resting tone and fetal heart rate changes; what is the priority intervention?
(A) Encourage deep breathing exercises
(B) Assist patient with ambulation
(C) Stop oxytocin and reposition patient
(D) Continue monitoring contraction pattern
Q536. A postpartum patient on day 3 reports breast fullness, warmth, and discomfort without fever or redness; what condition is most likely present?
(A) Hormonal imbalance state
(B) Vascular obstruction issue
(C) Breast engorgement state
(D) Infectious mastitis process
Q537. A newborn demonstrates a startle response with extension and abduction of arms followed by flexion when exposed to a sudden noise; what does this indicate?
(A) Normal neurological reflex
(B) Respiratory compromise
(C) Severe neurological deficit
(D) Feeding difficulty
Q538. A postpartum patient presents with a temperature of 38.4°C on day 4, along with uterine tenderness and foul-smelling lochia; how should this condition be interpreted?
(A) Normal postpartum response
(B) Uterine infection presence
(C) Hormonal adjustment phase
(D) Mild dehydration state
Q539. A newborn is placed skin-to-skin immediately after birth and maintains stable temperature and heart rate; what does this suggest about neonatal adaptation?
(A) Poor physiological stability
(B) Effective thermoregulation
(C) Circulatory compromise
(D) Increased metabolic stress

Q540. A multiparous patient presents to the labor unit stating contractions have been occurring every 2 minutes for the last hour, with inability to talk during contractions, increasing rectal pressure, and a strong urge to push; examination reveals full cervical dilation and fetal head at +3 station with visible crowning. What is the most appropriate immediate nursing action in this situation?
(A) Transfer patient for observation
(B) Encourage relaxation techniques
(C) Prepare for immediate delivery
(D) Delay pushing until provider arrives
Q541. A postpartum patient's uterus is firm and positioned 3 cm below the umbilicus on day 3; what does this indicate?
(A) Normal involution progress
(B) Delayed uterine recovery
(C) Retained placental tissue
(D) Early hemorrhage sign
Q542. A newborn turns the head toward a stimulus when the cheek is touched; what reflex is demonstrated?
(A) Moro reflex activity
(B) Grasp reflex action
(C) Tonic neck reflex
(D) Rooting reflex response
Q543. A patient in labor at 9 cm dilation experiences contractions every 2 minutes lasting 80 seconds with intense pressure; how should this stage be interpreted?
(A) Second stage labor
(B) Active labor phase
(C) Transition phase stage
(D) Latent phase stage
Q544. A postpartum patient experiences mild uterine cramping that increases during breastfeeding sessions; what is the physiological explanation for this finding?
(A) Fluid volume shift
(B) Estrogen level decline
(C) Progesterone withdrawal
(D) Oxytocin release effect
Q545. A laboring patient receiving oxytocin develops contractions every minute lasting over 90 seconds, and fetal heart rate shows late decelerations; what is the priority nursing intervention?
(A) Provide oral hydration
(B) Continue infusion monitoring
(C) Stop oxytocin and reposition
(D) Encourage pushing efforts
Q546. A postpartum patient on day 2 reports breast fullness and tightness without redness or fever; what condition is most likely present?
(A) Hormonal imbalance issue
(B) Infectious mastitis process
(C) Breast engorgement state
(D) Circulatory obstruction
Q547. A newborn exhibits a strong cry, active movement, and flexed posture shortly after birth; what does this indicate?
(A) Neurological impairment
(B) Effective neonatal adaptation

(C) Respiratory distress state
(D) Circulatory instability
Q548. A postpartum patient develops a temperature of 38.5°C on day 3 along with uterine tenderness and fatigue; how should this condition be interpreted?
(A) Hormonal fluctuation state
(B) Normal postpartum variation
(C) Uterine infection presence
(D) Mild dehydration effect
Q549. A newborn maintains stable vital signs including temperature, heart rate, and respiratory effort within the first hour after birth; what does this suggest?
(A) Delayed physiological adaptation
(B) Circulatory instability
(C) Successful neonatal transition
(D) Respiratory compromise
Q550. A multiparous patient presents to the labor unit stating contractions have been occurring every 2 minutes for over an hour, she is unable to talk during contractions, reports increasing rectal pressure and urge to push; examination reveals full dilation and fetal head at +3 station with crowning visible. What is the most appropriate immediate nursing action?
(A) Prepare for immediate delivery
(B) Delay pushing until reassessment
(C) Transfer patient to another unit
(D) Encourage relaxation techniques
Q551. A postpartum patient's uterus is firm and located midway between the umbilicus and symphysis pubis on day 4; what does this indicate?
(A) Early hemorrhage condition
(B) Normal uterine involution
(C) Delayed postpartum recovery
(D) Retained tissue presence
Q552. A newborn extends arms and legs symmetrically in response to sudden noise; what reflex is being demonstrated?
(A) Moro reflex response
(B) Grasp reflex activity
(C) Rooting reflex action
(D) Babinski reflex sign
Q553. A patient in labor at 3 cm dilation experiences contractions every 6 minutes lasting 40 seconds with mild discomfort; how should this labor stage be classified?
(A) Active phase labor
(B) Second stage labor
(C) Latent phase labor
(D) Transition phase stage
Q554. A postpartum patient reports passage of a small amount of dark blood after standing up from bed, and assessment reveals a firm uterus; what explains this finding?
(A) Infection development
(B) Coagulation disorder
(C) Uterine atony presence
(D) Normal pooled blood release
Q555. A laboring patient receiving oxytocin develops a contraction pattern of every 1 minute lasting 95 seconds with fetal heart rate showing late decelerations; what is the priority intervention?

(A) Provide oral hydration
(B) Continue infusion monitoring
(C) Encourage breathing exercises
(D) Stop oxytocin and reposition

Q556. A postpartum patient on day 3 reports breast fullness and mild discomfort without redness or fever; what is the most likely condition?
(A) Infectious mastitis process
(B) Breast engorgement state
(C) Circulatory obstruction
(D) Hormonal imbalance issue

Q557. A newborn demonstrates coordinated sucking, swallowing, and breathing during feeding; what does this indicate?
(A) Neurological deficit
(B) Gastrointestinal disorder
(C) Effective feeding ability
(D) Respiratory compromise

Q558. A postpartum patient presents with fever, uterine tenderness, and foul-smelling discharge on day 4 after delivery; how should this condition be interpreted?
(A) Hormonal fluctuation state
(B) Uterine infection presence
(C) Mild dehydration effect
(D) Normal postpartum variation

Q559. A newborn maintains stable temperature and respiratory effort during the first hour after birth without external warming support; what does this suggest?
(A) Circulatory compromise
(B) Increased metabolic stress
(C) Poor physiological stability
(D) Effective thermoregulation

Q560. A multiparous patient arrives reporting contractions every 2 minutes for over an hour, inability to speak during contractions, increasing rectal pressure, and a strong urge to push; examination reveals full cervical dilation, fetal head at +3 station, and visible crowning with perineal bulging. What is the most appropriate immediate nursing action in this situation?
(A) Encourage relaxation breathing
(B) Transfer patient for monitoring
(C) Delay pushing until provider arrives
(D) Prepare immediately for delivery

Q561. A postpartum patient's fundus is firm and located 4 cm below the umbilicus on day 4; what does this finding indicate?
(A) Normal involution progress
(B) Retained placental tissue
(C) Early hemorrhage condition
(D) Delayed uterine recovery

Q562. A newborn's feet appear bluish while the trunk remains pink during the first hours of life; what is this condition called?
(A) Severe hypoxia sign
(B) Peripheral acrocyanosis
(C) Central cyanosis state
(D) Circulatory failure

Q563. A laboring patient at 7 cm dilation has contractions every 2 minutes lasting 70 seconds with increasing pressure; how should this stage be interpreted?
(A) Active labor phase
(B) Latent phase stage
(C) Second stage labor
(D) Transition phase stage
Q564. A postpartum patient reports mild uterine cramping that becomes more noticeable during breastfeeding sessions; what explains this response?
(A) Fluid shift response
(B) Estrogen level decrease
(C) Oxytocin release effect
(D) Progesterone withdrawal
Q565. A laboring patient receiving oxytocin develops contractions every minute lasting 95 seconds with minimal relaxation, and fetal monitoring shows late decelerations; what is the priority intervention?
(A) Continue monitoring pattern
(B) Stop oxytocin and reposition
(C) Encourage breathing exercises
(D) Provide oral hydration
Q566. A postpartum patient on day 3 reports breast fullness, warmth, and mild discomfort without systemic symptoms; what condition is most likely present?
(A) Hormonal imbalance issue
(B) Infectious mastitis process
(C) Breast engorgement state
(D) Vascular obstruction
Q567. A newborn demonstrates a strong cry, flexed posture, and active movement immediately after birth; what does this indicate?
(A) Respiratory distress state
(B) Neurological impairment
(C) Circulatory instability
(D) Effective neonatal adaptation
Q568. A postpartum patient develops fever, uterine tenderness, and foul-smelling discharge on day 3 after delivery; how should this condition be interpreted?
(A) Mild dehydration effect
(B) Normal postpartum variation
(C) Uterine infection presence
(D) Hormonal fluctuation state
Q569. A newborn maintains stable temperature, heart rate, and respiratory effort without external warming support during the first hour; what does this suggest?
(A) Circulatory compromise
(B) Effective thermoregulation
(C) Poor physiological stability
(D) Increased metabolic stress
Q570. A multiparous patient arrives reporting contractions every 2 minutes for over an hour, inability to speak during contractions, increasing rectal pressure, and a strong urge to push; on examination, the cervix is fully dilated and the fetal head is at +3 station with visible crowning and bulging perineum. What is the most appropriate immediate nursing action?
(A) Encourage breathing techniques

(B) Prepare immediately for delivery
(C) Transfer patient for observation
(D) Delay pushing until provider arrives

Q571. A postpartum patient's uterus is firm and located halfway between the umbilicus and symphysis pubis on day 5; what does this indicate?
(A) Retained placental tissue
(B) Normal involution progress
(C) Early hemorrhage condition
(D) Delayed uterine recovery

Q572. A newborn's toes fan outward when the sole of the foot is stroked; what reflex is being demonstrated?
(A) Rooting reflex activity
(B) Babinski reflex response
(C) Moro reflex action
(D) Grasp reflex response

Q573. A laboring patient at 8 cm dilation reports very strong contractions every 2 minutes lasting 80 seconds, along with increasing pressure and irritability; how should this stage be interpreted?
(A) Active labor phase
(B) Transition phase stage
(C) Second stage labor
(D) Latent phase stage

Q574. A postpartum patient reports intermittent uterine cramping that intensifies during breastfeeding and gradually decreases afterward; what is the most appropriate explanation for this pattern?
(A) Progesterone imbalance
(B) Fluid redistribution
(C) Estrogen withdrawal effect
(D) Oxytocin-mediated contractions

Q575. A laboring patient receiving oxytocin develops a contraction pattern of every 1 minute lasting 100 seconds with minimal resting tone, and fetal monitoring shows repetitive late decelerations; what is the priority nursing intervention in this situation?
(A) Continue infusion monitoring
(B) Encourage breathing exercises
(C) Provide oral hydration
(D) Stop oxytocin and reposition

Q576. A postpartum patient on day 4 reports breast fullness with firm areas and mild discomfort but no fever, redness, or systemic symptoms; what condition is most likely present?
(A) Hormonal imbalance issue
(B) Breast engorgement state
(C) Infectious mastitis process
(D) Circulatory obstruction

Q577. A newborn exhibits a vigorous cry, flexed posture, active movement, and stable respiratory effort within minutes after birth; what does this indicate about neonatal adaptation?
(A) Circulatory instability
(B) Effective transition status
(C) Neurological impairment
(D) Respiratory distress state

Q578. A postpartum patient presents with a temperature of 38.6°C on day 3 along with uterine tenderness, fatigue, and foul-smelling lochia; how should this condition be interpreted?
(A) Mild dehydration effect
(B) Normal postpartum variation
(C) Hormonal fluctuation state
(D) Uterine infection presence
Q579. A newborn maintains stable body temperature, heart rate, and respiratory effort without the need for external warming devices during the first hour after birth; what does this suggest about the newborn's physiological status?
(A) Circulatory compromise
(B) Effective thermoregulation
(C) Poor physiological stability
(D) Increased metabolic stress
Q580. A multiparous patient arrives at the labor unit stating that contractions have been occurring every 2 minutes for the past hour, she is unable to speak during contractions, reports intense rectal pressure, and feels an overwhelming urge to push; upon examination, the cervix is fully dilated, the fetal head is at +3 station, and crowning with perineal bulging is observed. What is the most appropriate immediate nursing action in this situation?
(A) Encourage controlled breathing
(B) Prepare immediately for delivery
(C) Delay pushing until provider arrives
(D) Transfer patient for observation
Q581. A postpartum patient's fundus is firm and no longer palpable abdominally by day 10; what does this indicate?
(A) Early hemorrhage condition
(B) Normal involution completion
(C) Retained placental tissue
(D) Delayed uterine recovery
Q582. A newborn's trunk appears pink while the extremities remain slightly bluish during the first hours of life; what is this condition called?
(A) Central cyanosis state
(B) Circulatory collapse
(C) Peripheral acrocyanosis
(D) Severe hypoxia sign
Q583. A laboring patient at 6 cm dilation experiences contractions every 3 minutes lasting 60 seconds with moderate to strong intensity and increasing discomfort; how should this stage be interpreted?
(A) Transition phase stage
(B) Active labor phase
(C) Latent labor phase
(D) Second stage labor
Q584. A postpartum patient reports a sudden increase in vaginal bleeding after walking to the bathroom, but assessment reveals a firm, midline uterus and stable vital signs; what is the most appropriate interpretation of this finding?
(A) Uterine atony condition
(B) Coagulation disorder
(C) Normal pooled blood release
(D) Infection development

Q585. A laboring patient receiving oxytocin develops contractions every minute lasting 100 seconds with minimal resting tone, and fetal heart monitoring shows repetitive late decelerations with decreased variability; what is the priority nursing intervention in this situation?
(A) Provide oral hydration
(B) Continue infusion monitoring
(C) Stop oxytocin and reposition
(D) Encourage breathing exercises
Q586. A postpartum patient on day 4 reports breast fullness, firmness, and discomfort without fever, redness, or systemic symptoms, especially before feeding sessions; what condition is most likely present?
(A) Circulatory obstruction
(B) Breast engorgement state
(C) Hormonal imbalance issue
(D) Infectious mastitis process
Q587. A newborn exhibits a strong cry, active spontaneous movement, flexed posture, and stable respiratory effort within minutes after birth; what does this indicate about neonatal adaptation?
(A) Respiratory distress state
(B) Neurological impairment
(C) Circulatory instability
(D) Effective physiological transition
Q588. A postpartum patient presents on day 3 with a temperature of 38.7°C, uterine tenderness, fatigue, and foul-smelling lochia, along with mild tachycardia; how should this condition be interpreted?
(A) Mild dehydration effect
(B) Normal postpartum variation
(C) Hormonal fluctuation state
(D) Uterine infection presence
Q589. A newborn maintains stable body temperature, heart rate, and respiratory effort without external warming devices during the first hour after birth, while demonstrating active movement and normal tone; what does this suggest about neonatal physiological status?
(A) Effective thermoregulation
(B) Increased metabolic stress
(C) Poor physiological stability
(D) Circulatory compromise
Q590. A multiparous patient arrives at the labor unit reporting contractions every 2 minutes for the past hour, inability to speak during contractions, increasing rectal pressure, and a strong urge to push; on examination, the cervix is fully dilated, fetal head is at +3 station, and crowning with significant perineal bulging is observed, with the patient expressing inability to resist pushing. What is the most appropriate immediate nursing action in this situation?
(A) Delay pushing until provider arrives
(B) Encourage controlled breathing
(C) Transfer patient for monitoring
(D) Prepare immediately for delivery
Q591. A postpartum patient's uterus is no longer palpable abdominally and lochia has significantly decreased by day 10; what does this indicate?
(A) Normal involution completion
(B) Retained placental tissue
(C) Delayed uterine recovery

(D) Early hemorrhage condition

Q592. A newborn turns the head and opens the mouth when the cheek is touched; what reflex is demonstrated?

(A) Grasp reflex activity
(B) Rooting reflex response
(C) Moro reflex action
(D) Babinski reflex sign

Q593. A patient in labor at 5 cm dilation has contractions every 4 minutes lasting 55 seconds with moderate intensity and increasing discomfort; how should this stage be interpreted?

(A) Latent labor phase
(B) Transition phase stage
(C) Second stage labor
(D) Active labor phase

Q594. A postpartum patient reports noticing a small amount of dark red blood when standing after resting for several hours, but the uterus is firm and midline with stable vital signs; what is the most appropriate interpretation of this finding?

(A) Normal pooled blood release
(B) Uterine atony condition
(C) Coagulation disorder
(D) Infection development

Q595. A laboring patient receiving oxytocin develops contractions every minute lasting over 100 seconds with minimal resting tone, and fetal monitoring shows persistent late decelerations with decreased variability; what is the priority nursing intervention in this situation?

(A) Continue infusion monitoring
(B) Provide oral hydration
(C) Encourage breathing exercises
(D) Stop oxytocin and reposition

Q596. A postpartum patient on day 3 reports breast fullness, firmness, and discomfort that improves after feeding, with no fever or redness present; what condition is most likely present?

(A) Hormonal imbalance issue
(B) Infectious mastitis process
(C) Breast engorgement state
(D) Circulatory obstruction

Q597. A newborn exhibits strong cry, active movement, flexed posture, and stable respiratory effort shortly after birth; what does this indicate?

(A) Effective neonatal adaptation
(B) Circulatory instability
(C) Neurological impairment
(D) Respiratory distress state

Q598. A postpartum patient presents on day 4 with fever, uterine tenderness, foul-smelling lochia, and generalized fatigue, along with mild tachycardia; how should this condition be interpreted?

(A) Mild dehydration effect
(B) Normal postpartum variation
(C) Hormonal fluctuation state
(D) Uterine infection presence

Q599. A newborn maintains stable temperature, heart rate, and respiratory effort without external warming support during the first hour after birth, while demonstrating active movement and normal tone; what does this suggest about neonatal physiological status?

(A) Circulatory compromise
(B) Increased metabolic stress
(C) Effective thermoregulation
(D) Poor physiological stability

Q600. A multiparous patient arrives at the labor unit reporting contractions every 2 minutes for over an hour, inability to speak during contractions, increasing rectal pressure, and a strong urge to push; on examination, the cervix is fully dilated, the fetal head is at +3 station, and crowning with significant perineal bulging is observed, with the patient unable to resist pushing efforts. What is the most appropriate immediate nursing action in this situation?

(A) Prepare immediately for delivery
(B) Encourage controlled breathing
(C) Transfer patient for monitoring
(D) Delay pushing until provider arrives

Answer Key and Explanation (501-600)

Q501. Answer: B

Explanation: After delivery, the uterus gradually descends approximately one fingerbreadth per day. A firm fundus below the umbilicus on day one indicates proper involution. This suggests effective contraction and reduced bleeding risk. Regular assessment ensures continued downward progression. Any deviation from this pattern may require evaluation. This finding supports a normal postpartum recovery process. ##

Q502. Answer: D

Explanation: Acrocyanosis refers to bluish discoloration of the extremities while the central body remains pink. This occurs due to immature peripheral circulation in newborns. It is a common and temporary finding shortly after birth. The condition resolves as circulation stabilizes. Continuous observation ensures no progression to central cyanosis. This is considered a normal transitional response. ##

Q503. Answer: B

Explanation: At 5 cm dilation with moderate contractions, the patient is in the active phase of labor. This phase involves progressive cervical dilation and increasing contraction intensity. The pattern indicates effective labor progression. Pain levels typically increase as dilation advances. Monitoring ensures both maternal and fetal well-being. This stage leads toward full dilation. ##

Q504. Answer: B

Explanation: Increased bleeding after movement can occur due to pooled blood being expelled. A firm uterus indicates that uterine tone is adequate. This suggests that active hemorrhage is not occurring. Monitoring the amount and frequency of bleeding remains important. The finding is common during early ambulation. It generally does not indicate a complication if transient. ##

Q505. Answer: B

Explanation: Excessively frequent and prolonged contractions indicate uterine tachysystole. This can compromise fetal oxygenation by reducing placental blood flow. Discontinuing oxytocin is the first step to reduce uterine activity. Continuous monitoring is required to assess recovery. Additional interventions may be needed if the pattern persists. Prompt action prevents fetal distress. ##

Q506. Answer: C

Explanation: Localized breast pain with redness and fever indicates an infectious process. This commonly results from bacterial entry through cracked nipples. Milk stasis can contribute to the development of inflammation. Early treatment with antibiotics is important. Continued breastfeeding helps maintain milk flow. Prompt care prevents complications such as abscess formation. ##

Q507. Answer: C

Explanation: A strong suck reflex and coordinated swallowing indicate proper neurological function. These abilities are essential for effective feeding. The coordination reflects intact cranial nerve function. Assessment of feeding behaviors is part of routine newborn evaluation. Consistent feeding patterns support adequate nutrition. This finding is a sign of healthy development. ##

Q508. Answer: A

Explanation: A mild temperature elevation within the first 24 hours postpartum can be a normal response. It is often related to dehydration or exertion during labor. Absence of additional symptoms reduces concern for infection. Monitoring temperature trends is important. Persistent fever would require further evaluation. This finding is generally self-limiting. ##

Q509. Answer: D

Explanation: Skin-to-skin contact helps regulate the newborn's temperature effectively. It reduces heat loss and stabilizes vital signs. This practice also supports early bonding and breastfeeding. Maintaining thermal stability decreases metabolic stress. Continuous observation ensures safety during this period. It is a key component of immediate newborn care. ##

Q510. Answer: C

Explanation: Full cervical dilation with fetal descent and urge to push indicates the second stage of labor. A +2 station confirms that the fetus is well into the birth canal. Immediate preparation for delivery is necessary to ensure safety. Rapid progression is common in multiparous patients. Continuous support and monitoring are essential. This situation requires prompt readiness for birth. ##

Q511. Answer: C

Explanation: Immediately after delivery, the uterus is expected to be firm and positioned at the level of the umbilicus. This indicates effective uterine contraction and reduced risk of hemorrhage. Proper tone helps compress blood vessels and control bleeding. Continuous monitoring ensures that the uterus remains firm. Any softening or displacement would require intervention. This finding reflects a stable postpartum condition. ##

Q512. Answer: D

Explanation: The rooting reflex helps the newborn locate the breast or feeding source. When the cheek is touched, the infant turns toward the stimulus. This behavior is essential for successful feeding. It reflects intact neurological function. The reflex is present at birth and fades over time. It supports early nutritional intake and bonding. ##

Q513. Answer: C

Explanation: At 6 cm dilation with regular, strong contractions, the patient is in active labor. This phase involves faster cervical dilation and increased contraction intensity. The pattern indicates effective labor progression. Pain typically intensifies during this stage. Monitoring ensures fetal well-being and maternal safety. This phase leads toward complete dilation. ##

Q514. Answer: A

Explanation: After lying down, blood may collect in the vagina and be released upon standing. A firm uterus indicates adequate contraction and control of bleeding. This suggests that the bleeding is not due to hemorrhage. Monitoring the amount and frequency remains important. This occurrence is common in early postpartum recovery. It is generally considered a normal finding. ##

Q515. Answer: D

Explanation: Excessive uterine activity reduces blood flow to the fetus. Stopping oxytocin decreases contraction frequency and intensity. Repositioning improves maternal circulation and placental perfusion. Continuous monitoring evaluates fetal response. Additional measures may be required if distress persists. Early intervention prevents worsening hypoxia. ##

Q516. Answer: B

Explanation: Breast engorgement occurs when milk production exceeds removal. This leads to swelling, firmness, and discomfort. It is common in the early postpartum period as milk supply increases. Frequent feeding or expression helps relieve symptoms. Monitoring ensures no progression to infection. This condition reflects a normal physiological adjustment. ##

Q517. Answer: A

Explanation: Strong cry, active movement, and good tone are indicators of effective adaptation. These signs reflect proper respiratory and neurological function. Adequate oxygenation supports normal activity levels. Continuous monitoring confirms stability. These findings are expected in healthy newborns. They indicate successful transition to extrauterine life. ##

Q518. Answer: C

Explanation: Persistent fever with uterine tenderness suggests infection of the uterine lining. This condition often develops within a few days postpartum. Symptoms such as malaise indicate systemic involvement. Early antibiotic treatment is necessary to control the infection. Monitoring vital signs helps assess progression. Prompt management reduces complications. ##

Q519. Answer: A
Explanation: Stable temperature and oxygen saturation indicate effective neonatal adaptation. The newborn is maintaining physiological balance with minimal support. Proper thermoregulation reduces metabolic demand. Adequate oxygenation supports organ function. Continuous monitoring ensures sustained stability. This reflects a healthy transition period. ##
Q520. Answer: D
Explanation: Full dilation with fetal head at +3 station indicates imminent birth. Strong urge to push confirms entry into the second stage of labor. Rapid progression is common in multiparous patients. Immediate preparation ensures safe delivery conditions. Continuous monitoring of fetal status is essential. Prompt readiness reduces risk of complications during birth. ##
Q521. Answer: C
Explanation: Lochia serosa typically appears a few days after delivery as bleeding decreases. A firm uterus indicates effective contraction and proper involution. The reduced amount of discharge suggests normal healing progression. Monitoring ensures no abnormal increase or foul odor develops. This pattern reflects expected postpartum recovery. Continued assessment confirms stability over time. ##
Q522. Answer: D
Explanation: The Moro reflex is a normal response to sudden stimuli in newborns. It reflects proper functioning of the central nervous system. The reflex includes arm extension followed by flexion. Its presence indicates intact neurological pathways. Absence or asymmetry may suggest underlying issues. This finding supports normal neonatal development. ##
Q523. Answer: B
Explanation: Cervical dilation of 8 cm with very strong and frequent contractions indicates transition phase. This is the final part of the first stage of labor. Intensity and frequency of contractions peak during this stage. Patients often experience increased discomfort and pressure. Close monitoring is essential for safety. This phase precedes full dilation and pushing. ##
Q524. Answer: A
Explanation: Breastfeeding stimulates oxytocin release, which increases uterine contractions. These contractions can temporarily increase bleeding as the uterus expels contents. A firm and midline uterus indicates adequate tone. This suggests that the bleeding is controlled and expected. Monitoring ensures the bleeding does not become excessive. This is a normal physiological response. ##
Q525. Answer: C
Explanation: Excessive uterine contractions reduce oxygen delivery to the fetus. Stopping oxytocin helps decrease contraction frequency and intensity. This intervention improves uteroplacental blood flow. Continuous monitoring is necessary to assess recovery. Additional supportive measures may be required. Prompt action prevents worsening fetal compromise. ##
Q526. Answer: B
Explanation: Breast engorgement occurs due to accumulation of milk in the breast tissue. It often presents with firmness and discomfort but no systemic symptoms. This condition is common during early lactation. Frequent feeding or pumping helps relieve symptoms. Monitoring ensures it does not progress to infection. It represents a normal adjustment process. ##
Q527. Answer: A
Explanation: Coordinated suck, swallow, and breathing are essential for effective feeding. This coordination indicates proper neurological and muscular function. It ensures safe intake of nutrition without aspiration. Consistent feeding patterns support growth and development. Monitoring confirms sustained coordination. This finding reflects healthy neonatal adaptation. ##
Q528. Answer: A
Explanation: Fever combined with uterine tenderness suggests an infectious process. This commonly involves the uterine lining after delivery. Symptoms appearing after the first 24 hours raise concern for

infection. Early antibiotic therapy is necessary to manage the condition. Monitoring helps track response to treatment. Prompt care prevents complications. ##

Q529. Answer: B

Explanation: Stable vital signs indicate effective adaptation to extrauterine life. The newborn is maintaining physiological balance independently. Proper temperature control reduces metabolic stress. Adequate respiratory effort ensures oxygenation. Continuous monitoring confirms stability. This finding reflects a healthy transition process. ##

Q530. Answer: B

Explanation: Full dilation with crowning indicates that birth is imminent. The fetal head at +3 station confirms advanced descent. Strong urge to push reflects second stage of labor. Immediate preparation ensures safe and timely delivery. Continuous monitoring supports maternal and fetal safety. Rapid action reduces risk of complications. ##

Q531. Answer: A

Explanation: The uterus normally descends about 1 to 2 cm each day after delivery. A position below the umbilicus on day two reflects appropriate involution. Firmness indicates effective contraction and reduced bleeding risk. This progression shows that the uterus is returning to its pre-pregnancy size. Regular assessment confirms continued downward movement. This finding is consistent with normal postpartum recovery. ##

Q532. Answer: D

Explanation: The palmar grasp reflex is a normal newborn reflex present at birth. It demonstrates intact neurological pathways and muscle tone. When stimulated, the infant closes the hand around the object. This reflex gradually disappears as voluntary control develops. Its presence is part of routine neonatal assessment. It indicates normal neurological function. ##

Q533. Answer: D

Explanation: Contractions that are mild and spaced apart indicate the latent phase of labor. Cervical dilation at 4 cm supports this classification. Progression during this phase is gradual. Discomfort is usually manageable compared to later stages. Monitoring ensures labor continues to progress appropriately. This phase precedes active labor. ##

Q534. Answer: B

Explanation: Blood can accumulate in the vaginal canal while the patient is lying down. Upon standing, this pooled blood is released, causing a temporary increase in bleeding. A firm and midline uterus indicates adequate contraction and control. This confirms that the bleeding is not due to hemorrhage. Monitoring ensures the amount remains within expected limits. This is a common and normal postpartum occurrence. ##

Q535. Answer: C

Explanation: Excessively frequent contractions reduce oxygen delivery to the fetus. Discontinuing oxytocin decreases uterine stimulation. Repositioning improves maternal circulation and placental perfusion. Continuous monitoring is required to assess fetal recovery. Additional interventions may be necessary if the condition persists. Prompt action is essential to prevent fetal distress. ##

Q536. Answer: C

Explanation: Breast engorgement occurs when milk production exceeds removal. It results in fullness, warmth, and discomfort. The absence of fever or redness helps differentiate it from infection. Frequent breastfeeding or pumping helps relieve symptoms. Monitoring ensures no progression to mastitis. This condition is a normal part of early lactation. ##

Q537. Answer: A

Explanation: This description represents the Moro reflex, a normal newborn response. It indicates proper neurological function and central nervous system integrity. The reflex is triggered by sudden stimuli such as noise or movement. It is present at birth and fades over time. Assessment ensures symmetry and presence. This finding supports healthy neurological development. ##

Q538. Answer: B

Explanation: Fever with uterine tenderness and foul-smelling discharge indicates infection. This condition commonly affects the uterine lining after delivery. Symptoms appearing after the first 24 hours raise concern for infection. Early antibiotic treatment is required to control the condition. Monitoring ensures response to therapy. Prompt management prevents complications. ##

Q539. Answer: B

Explanation: Skin-to-skin contact helps maintain body temperature in newborns. Stable vital signs indicate effective adaptation to the external environment. This reduces the risk of hypothermia and metabolic stress. The newborn is able to maintain physiological balance. Continuous monitoring ensures ongoing stability. This reflects successful early neonatal transition. ##

Q540. Answer: C

Explanation: Full cervical dilation combined with crowning indicates that delivery is imminent. The fetal head at +3 station confirms advanced descent into the birth canal. Strong urge to push is consistent with second stage labor. Immediate preparation ensures safe and timely delivery. Continuous monitoring supports maternal and fetal safety. Rapid response minimizes risk of complications. ##

Q541. Answer: A

Explanation: The uterus typically descends approximately 1 to 2 cm per day after delivery. A position 3 cm below the umbilicus on day three reflects expected involution. Firmness indicates effective contraction and control of bleeding. This pattern demonstrates proper healing and recovery. Continuous monitoring ensures consistent progression. This finding supports a normal postpartum course. ##

Q542. Answer: D

Explanation: The rooting reflex helps the newborn locate a source of feeding. When the cheek is stimulated, the infant turns toward the touch. This reflex is essential for successful breastfeeding. It indicates intact neurological pathways. The reflex is present at birth and fades over time. It supports early feeding behaviors. ##

Q543. Answer: C

Explanation: Cervical dilation of 9 cm with strong and frequent contractions indicates transition phase. This is the final part of the first stage of labor. Intensity of contractions reaches its peak during this stage. Patients often feel increased pressure and discomfort. Close monitoring is required for maternal and fetal safety. This stage precedes full dilation and delivery. ##

Q544. Answer: D

Explanation: Breastfeeding stimulates the release of oxytocin from the posterior pituitary. This hormone causes uterine contractions that help reduce uterine size. These contractions also assist in minimizing postpartum bleeding. The increased cramping during feeding is a normal response. Over time, the discomfort typically decreases. This process supports effective uterine involution. ##

Q545. Answer: C

Explanation: Excessive uterine activity reduces placental blood flow and fetal oxygenation. Discontinuing oxytocin helps decrease contraction frequency. Repositioning improves circulation and oxygen delivery to the fetus. Continuous monitoring is essential to evaluate response. Additional interventions may be required if the condition persists. Prompt action is necessary to prevent fetal compromise. ##

Q546. Answer: C

Explanation: Breast engorgement occurs when milk production increases and accumulates. It leads to fullness, tightness, and discomfort. The absence of fever or redness helps differentiate it from infection. Frequent feeding or pumping helps relieve symptoms. Monitoring ensures the condition does not worsen. This is a normal early postpartum change. ##

Q547. Answer: B

Explanation: A strong cry and active movement indicate good oxygenation and neurological function. Flexed posture reflects normal muscle tone in newborns. These findings are signs of successful adaptation to extrauterine life. Continuous monitoring ensures stability is maintained. These indicators are expected in healthy infants. This reflects normal neonatal transition. ##

Q548. Answer: C

Explanation: Fever with uterine tenderness suggests infection of the uterine lining. Symptoms appearing after the first 24 hours are concerning for infection. Fatigue may indicate systemic involvement. Early antibiotic therapy is essential for treatment. Monitoring helps assess response to therapy. Prompt intervention prevents complications. ##

Q549. Answer: C

Explanation: Stable vital signs indicate effective adaptation to the external environment. The newborn is maintaining physiological balance independently. Proper thermoregulation and oxygenation are established. Continuous monitoring ensures ongoing stability. These findings are expected in healthy newborns. This reflects a successful transition period. ##

Q550. Answer: A

Explanation: Full cervical dilation with crowning indicates that birth is imminent. The fetal head at +3 station confirms advanced descent. Strong urge to push is consistent with the second stage of labor. Immediate preparation ensures safe delivery conditions. Continuous monitoring supports both maternal and fetal safety. Rapid response minimizes risk of complications. ##

Q551. Answer: B

Explanation: The uterus continues to descend daily after delivery as part of involution. By day four, it is expected to be positioned below the umbilicus toward the symphysis pubis. Firmness indicates effective contraction and reduced bleeding risk. This gradual descent reflects proper healing and recovery. Regular assessment ensures continued normal progression. This finding is consistent with expected postpartum physiology. ##

Q552. Answer: A

Explanation: The Moro reflex is triggered by sudden stimuli such as loud noise. It involves extension and abduction of limbs followed by flexion. This reflex indicates intact neurological pathways. It is present at birth and gradually disappears over time. Symmetry is important for normal assessment. Its presence reflects normal neonatal neurological function. ##

Q553. Answer: C

Explanation: Mild contractions with longer intervals indicate the latent phase of labor. Cervical dilation at 3 cm supports early labor classification. Progression during this phase is gradual and may vary in duration. Discomfort is usually manageable. Monitoring ensures that labor continues to progress normally. This stage precedes active labor. ##

Q554. Answer: D

Explanation: Blood may collect in the vaginal canal while lying down. When the patient stands, this pooled blood is expelled. A firm uterus indicates effective contraction and control of bleeding. This confirms that the finding is not due to hemorrhage. Monitoring ensures the amount remains within expected limits. This is a common and normal postpartum occurrence. ##

Q555. Answer: D

Explanation: Excessive contraction frequency reduces placental blood flow. Late decelerations indicate decreased fetal oxygenation. Discontinuing oxytocin decreases uterine stimulation. Repositioning improves maternal circulation and oxygen delivery. Continuous monitoring is required to assess improvement. Prompt intervention is essential to prevent fetal compromise. ##

Q556. Answer: B

Explanation: Breast engorgement occurs when milk accumulates in the breast tissue. It leads to fullness and discomfort but lacks signs of infection. This condition is common during early lactation. Frequent feeding or pumping helps relieve symptoms. Monitoring ensures no progression to infection. It represents a normal physiological adjustment. ##

Q557. Answer: C

Explanation: Coordination of sucking, swallowing, and breathing is essential for feeding. This indicates intact neurological and muscular function. Proper coordination prevents aspiration and ensures adequate nutrition. Assessment of feeding behaviors is part of routine care. Consistent patterns support growth and development. This finding reflects normal neonatal adaptation. ##

Q558. Answer: B

Explanation: Fever with uterine tenderness and foul discharge indicates infection of the uterine lining. Symptoms appearing after the first 24 hours raise concern for infection. Early diagnosis is important for effective treatment. Antibiotic therapy is typically required. Monitoring ensures response to treatment. Prompt intervention prevents complications. ##

Q559. Answer: D

Explanation: Maintaining stable temperature without assistance indicates effective thermoregulation. The newborn is adapting well to the external environment. Proper temperature control reduces metabolic demand. Adequate respiratory effort supports oxygenation. Continuous monitoring ensures stability is maintained. This reflects successful neonatal transition. ##

Q560. Answer: D

Explanation: Full dilation with crowning indicates that delivery is imminent. The fetal head at +3 station confirms advanced descent. Strong urge to push reflects second stage labor. Immediate preparation ensures safe delivery conditions. Continuous monitoring supports maternal and fetal safety. Rapid action reduces risk of complications during birth. ##

Q561. Answer: A

Explanation: The uterus typically descends approximately one centimeter per day after delivery. A position 4 cm below the umbilicus on day four reflects expected involution. Firmness indicates adequate uterine contraction and control of bleeding. This pattern shows proper postpartum healing. Continuous monitoring ensures consistent progression. This finding is within normal recovery expectations. ##

Q562. Answer: B

Explanation: Acrocyanosis refers to bluish discoloration of the extremities in newborns. It occurs due to immature peripheral circulation. The central body remaining pink indicates adequate oxygenation. This finding is common and temporary in early life. It resolves as circulation stabilizes. This is considered a normal transitional response. ##

Q563. Answer: A

Explanation: Cervical dilation of 7 cm with strong, frequent contractions indicates active labor. This stage involves rapid cervical change and increased contraction intensity. The contraction pattern supports effective progression. Pressure increases as the fetus descends. Monitoring ensures maternal and fetal safety. This phase leads into transition. ##

Q564. Answer: C

Explanation: Breastfeeding stimulates oxytocin release, causing uterine contractions. These contractions help the uterus return to its pre-pregnancy size. The increased cramping during feeding is expected. This process also helps reduce postpartum bleeding. The discomfort usually decreases over time. It represents a normal physiological mechanism. ##

Q565. Answer: B

Explanation: Excessive contractions reduce uteroplacental blood flow and fetal oxygenation. Late decelerations indicate fetal distress related to hypoxia. Stopping oxytocin decreases contraction frequency. Repositioning improves circulation and oxygen delivery. Continuous monitoring evaluates recovery. Prompt intervention is critical to prevent complications. ##

Q566. Answer: C

Explanation: Breast engorgement occurs when milk accumulates in the breast tissue. It causes fullness, warmth, and discomfort. The absence of fever or redness distinguishes it from infection. Frequent feeding or pumping relieves symptoms. Monitoring ensures it does not progress. This is a normal postpartum condition. ##

Q567. Answer: D

Explanation: A strong cry indicates good lung expansion and oxygenation. Flexed posture reflects normal muscle tone. Active movement shows intact neurological function. These findings are consistent with a healthy newborn. Continuous monitoring ensures stability. This reflects successful adaptation to extrauterine life. ##

Q568. Answer: C

Explanation: Fever with uterine tenderness suggests infection of the uterine lining. Foul-smelling discharge further supports this diagnosis. Symptoms after the first 24 hours raise concern. Early antibiotic therapy is necessary. Monitoring helps assess response to treatment. Prompt management prevents complications. ##

Q569. Answer: B

Explanation: Maintaining stable temperature without assistance indicates proper thermoregulation. The newborn is adapting well to the environment. Adequate respiratory effort supports oxygenation. Stable heart rate reflects circulatory stability. Continuous monitoring ensures ongoing balance. This indicates successful neonatal transition. ##

Q570. Answer: B

Explanation: Full cervical dilation with crowning indicates imminent delivery. The fetal head at +3 station confirms advanced descent. Strong urge to push is characteristic of second stage labor. Immediate preparation ensures safety for both mother and newborn. Continuous monitoring supports optimal outcomes. Rapid response minimizes complications during delivery. ##

Q571. Answer: B

Explanation: The uterus continues to descend steadily after delivery as part of involution. By day five, it is expected to be well below the umbilicus. A firm uterus indicates adequate contraction and reduced bleeding risk. This pattern reflects normal healing and recovery. Regular monitoring ensures continued progression. This finding is consistent with expected postpartum physiology. ##

Q572. Answer: B

Explanation: The Babinski reflex is present in newborns due to immature nervous system development. Stroking the sole causes the toes to fan outward. This response is normal in infants but abnormal in adults. It indicates intact neurological pathways. The reflex disappears as the nervous system matures. Its presence supports normal neonatal development. ##

Q573. Answer: B

Explanation: Cervical dilation of 8 cm with intense, frequent contractions indicates the transition phase. This is the final part of the first stage of labor. Contractions become stronger and closer together during this stage. Patients often feel increased pressure and emotional changes. Monitoring is essential for maternal and fetal safety. This phase precedes full dilation. ##

Q574. Answer: D

Explanation: Breastfeeding stimulates the release of oxytocin, which causes uterine contractions. These contractions help the uterus shrink and return to its normal size. The increase in cramping during feeding is expected due to hormone release. This process also aids in reducing postpartum bleeding. The discomfort typically lessens over time. It reflects a normal physiological mechanism supporting recovery. ##

Q575. Answer: D

Explanation: Excessive uterine contractions reduce blood flow to the placenta. This leads to decreased oxygen delivery to the fetus. Late decelerations indicate fetal hypoxia. Discontinuing oxytocin helps reduce contraction frequency. Repositioning improves maternal circulation and oxygenation. Immediate intervention is necessary to prevent fetal compromise. ##

Q576. Answer: B

Explanation: Breast engorgement occurs when milk accumulates in the breast tissue. It results in firmness, fullness, and discomfort. The absence of systemic symptoms helps differentiate it from infection. Frequent feeding or pumping can relieve the condition. Monitoring ensures it does not progress to mastitis. This is a common and normal postpartum occurrence. ##

Q577. Answer: B

Explanation: A vigorous cry indicates strong respiratory effort and adequate oxygenation. Flexed posture reflects normal muscle tone. Active movement shows intact neurological function. Stable respiration confirms effective lung adaptation. These findings together indicate successful transition. Continuous monitoring ensures ongoing stability. ##

Q578. Answer: D

Explanation: Fever combined with uterine tenderness suggests infection of the uterine lining. Foul-smelling lochia further supports this diagnosis. Symptoms after the first 24 hours are concerning. Early antibiotic therapy is essential for treatment. Monitoring ensures response to therapy. Prompt intervention prevents complications. ##

Q579. Answer: B

Explanation: Stable temperature without external support indicates effective thermoregulation. The newborn is adapting well to the external environment. Proper temperature control reduces metabolic demand. Adequate respiratory effort supports oxygenation. Continuous monitoring ensures stability. This reflects successful neonatal adaptation. ##

Q580. Answer: B

Explanation: Full cervical dilation with crowning indicates that delivery is imminent. The fetal head at +3 station confirms advanced descent into the birth canal. Strong urge to push reflects second stage labor. Immediate preparation ensures safe and timely delivery. Continuous monitoring supports maternal and fetal safety. Rapid intervention minimizes risk of complications. ##

Q581. Answer: B

Explanation: By approximately 10 days postpartum, the uterus descends into the pelvic cavity. At this point, it is no longer palpable abdominally. This indicates near completion of involution. A firm uterus suggests adequate contraction and healing. Regular assessments confirm expected recovery. This finding reflects normal postpartum physiology. ##

Q582. Answer: C

Explanation: Acrocyanosis is a common finding in newborns due to immature peripheral circulation. The trunk remains pink, indicating adequate oxygenation. The bluish discoloration is limited to hands and feet. This condition resolves as circulation stabilizes. It does not indicate respiratory compromise. This is a normal transitional finding. ##

Q583. Answer: B

Explanation: Cervical dilation of 6 cm with regular, strong contractions indicates active labor. This stage is marked by faster cervical change. Contraction intensity and frequency increase progressively. The patient's discomfort typically intensifies. Monitoring ensures continued progression and safety. This phase leads toward transition. ##

Q584. Answer: C

Explanation: Blood can pool in the vaginal canal when the patient is lying down. Movement causes this collected blood to be expelled suddenly. A firm uterus indicates proper contraction and control of bleeding. Stable vital signs further support a non-emergent situation. Monitoring ensures that bleeding remains within normal limits. This is a common postpartum occurrence. ##

Q585. Answer: C

Explanation: Excessive uterine activity decreases placental blood flow. This leads to reduced oxygen delivery to the fetus. Late decelerations with decreased variability indicate fetal distress. Discontinuing oxytocin reduces contraction frequency. Repositioning improves maternal circulation and oxygenation. Immediate action is necessary to prevent fetal compromise. ##

Q586. Answer: B

Explanation: Breast engorgement occurs when milk accumulates in the breast tissue. It leads to fullness, firmness, and discomfort. The absence of fever and redness helps distinguish it from infection. Symptoms often improve after feeding or expression. Monitoring ensures no progression to mastitis. This condition is common in early lactation. ##

Q587. Answer: D

Explanation: A strong cry indicates good lung expansion and oxygenation. Active movement reflects intact neurological function. Flexed posture is a sign of normal muscle tone. Stable respiratory effort confirms effective adaptation. These findings collectively indicate a healthy newborn. Continuous monitoring ensures stability. ##

Q588. Answer: D

Explanation: Fever with uterine tenderness and foul discharge indicates infection of the uterine lining. Tachycardia suggests systemic involvement. Symptoms appearing after the first 24 hours are concerning. Early antibiotic therapy is required to treat the infection. Monitoring ensures response to treatment. Prompt management prevents further complications. ##

Q589. Answer: A

Explanation: Stable temperature without assistance indicates effective thermoregulation. Normal heart rate and respiration reflect adequate adaptation. Active movement and tone suggest intact neurological function. These findings indicate balanced physiological status. Continuous monitoring ensures stability is maintained. This reflects successful neonatal transition. ##

Q590. Answer: D

Explanation: Full cervical dilation with crowning indicates imminent delivery. The fetal head at +3 station confirms advanced descent. Strong urge to push reflects second stage labor. Immediate preparation ensures safe and timely birth. Continuous monitoring supports maternal and fetal safety. Rapid response minimizes complications during delivery. ##

Q591. Answer: A

Explanation: By around day ten postpartum, the uterus descends into the pelvic cavity and is no longer palpable. This marks near completion of involution. Decreased lochia indicates reduced shedding of the uterine lining. These findings together reflect appropriate healing. Continued monitoring ensures no abnormal symptoms develop. This is consistent with normal postpartum recovery. ##

Q592. Answer: B

Explanation: The rooting reflex helps the newborn locate a food source. Stimulation of the cheek triggers head turning and mouth opening. This reflex supports effective feeding behavior. It is present at birth and fades with neurological maturation. Assessment of this reflex is part of routine newborn evaluation. Its presence indicates normal neurological function. ##

Q593. Answer: D

Explanation: Cervical dilation at 5 cm with regular contractions indicates active labor. This stage involves more rapid cervical change. Contractions become stronger and more frequent. The patient experiences increasing discomfort. Monitoring ensures labor progression continues appropriately. This phase leads toward transition. ##

Q594. Answer: A

Explanation: Blood can collect in the vaginal canal while the patient is lying down. When standing, this pooled blood may be released suddenly. A firm uterus indicates effective contraction and control of bleeding. Stable vital signs further support a non-emergent condition. Monitoring ensures bleeding remains within expected limits. This is a common postpartum occurrence. ##

Q595. Answer: D

Explanation: Excessive uterine contractions reduce placental blood flow. This leads to decreased oxygen delivery to the fetus. Late decelerations with decreased variability indicate fetal distress. Stopping oxytocin reduces contraction frequency. Repositioning improves circulation and oxygenation. Immediate action is essential to prevent fetal compromise. ##

Q596. Answer: C

Explanation: Breast engorgement occurs due to accumulation of milk in the breast tissue. It leads to fullness, firmness, and discomfort. Improvement after feeding supports this diagnosis. The absence of fever or redness distinguishes it from infection. Monitoring ensures it does not progress to mastitis. This is a normal postpartum condition. ##

Q597. Answer: A

Explanation: A strong cry indicates effective lung expansion and oxygenation. Active movement reflects intact neurological function. Flexed posture shows normal muscle tone. Stable respiratory effort confirms adequate adaptation. These findings indicate a healthy newborn. Continuous monitoring ensures ongoing stability. ##

Q598. Answer: D

Explanation: Fever with uterine tenderness suggests infection of the uterine lining. Foul-smelling lochia supports this diagnosis. Tachycardia indicates systemic involvement. Symptoms after the first 24 hours are concerning. Early antibiotic therapy is required. Prompt management prevents complications. ##

Q599. Answer: C

Explanation: Stable temperature without assistance indicates effective thermoregulation. Normal heart rate and respiration reflect good adaptation. Active movement and tone show intact neurological function. These findings indicate balanced physiological status. Continuous monitoring ensures stability. This reflects successful neonatal transition. ##

Q600. Answer: A

Explanation: Full cervical dilation with crowning indicates that delivery is imminent. The fetal head at +3 station confirms advanced descent. Strong urge to push reflects second stage labor. Immediate preparation ensures safe and timely birth. Continuous monitoring supports maternal and fetal safety. Rapid response minimizes complications. ## Question (601-700)

Question (601-700)

Q601. The hormone responsible for the milk ejection reflex during breastfeeding is what?
(A) Oxytocin hormone release
(B) Progesterone hormone action
(C) Estrogen hormone activity
(D) Prolactin hormone release

Q602. A postpartum patient is preparing for discharge and asks how often breastfeeding should occur in the early weeks; what is the correct recommendation?
(A) Feed on demand frequently
(B) Feed every 6 hours
(C) Feed every 8 hours
(D) Feed once at night

Q603. A postpartum patient reports cracked nipples and pain during breastfeeding, especially at latch initiation, and states the infant frequently slips off the breast; what is the most appropriate nursing intervention?
(A) Suggest switching to bottle feeding
(B) Advise stopping breastfeeding temporarily
(C) Recommend decreasing feeding frequency
(D) Evaluate latch technique and positioning

Q604. A newborn develops jitteriness, poor feeding, and irritability within hours after birth, and blood glucose is found to be low; what condition is most likely present?
(A) Neonatal hypoglycemia state
(B) Neonatal infection process
(C) Respiratory distress syndrome
(D) Thermoregulation failure

Q605. A newborn fails to initiate breathing immediately after birth, has poor muscle tone, and a heart rate below 100 beats per minute; what is the priority initial intervention?
(A) Administer epinephrine
(B) Delay intervention briefly
(C) Begin positive pressure ventilation
(D) Start chest compressions

Q606. A postpartum patient reports feeling overwhelmed, tearful, and emotionally labile on day 3 after delivery but denies thoughts of harm; what condition is most likely present?
(A) Anxiety disorder
(B) Postpartum depression
(C) Psychotic disorder
(D) Postpartum blues condition

Q607. A newborn is noted to have a temperature below normal range shortly after birth despite appropriate clothing and environment; what is the most likely complication?
(A) Neonatal hypothermia state
(B) Respiratory distress
(C) Neonatal hyperthermia
(D) Infection presence

Q608. A postpartum patient develops unilateral leg swelling, warmth, pain, and redness on day 5 after delivery, especially with ambulation; what condition should be suspected?
(A) Deep vein thrombosis
(B) Fluid retention state

(C) Normal postpartum edema
(D) Muscle strain injury

Q609. A newborn requires stimulation at birth, has a weak cry, decreased muscle tone, and a heart rate just above 100 beats per minute but improves with minimal intervention; what does this indicate about neonatal transition?

(A) Mild adaptation difficulty
(B) Circulatory collapse
(C) Severe respiratory failure
(D) Neurological impairment

Q610. A postpartum patient preparing for discharge states she plans to stop breastfeeding because she believes formula is easier, expresses concern about returning to work, and reports limited family support; the nurse assesses knowledge gaps and emotional concerns. What is the most appropriate nursing action in this situation?

(A) Avoid discussing feeding choices
(B) Encourage immediate formula use
(C) Advise discontinuing breastfeeding
(D) Provide education and support resources

Q611. Colostrum is produced during the early postpartum period and is best described as what type of milk?

(A) Low protein secretion
(B) Thick antibody-rich milk
(C) High fat mature milk
(D) Diluted transitional milk

Q612. A newborn requires resuscitation and has a heart rate below 60 beats per minute after adequate ventilation; what is the next step in management?

(A) Administer oxygen only
(B) Continue observation only
(C) Provide oral feeding
(D) Begin chest compressions

Q613. A postpartum patient reports breast pain, localized redness, fever, and flu-like symptoms while breastfeeding on day 6; what is the most appropriate nursing intervention?

(A) Recommend formula substitution
(B) Stop breastfeeding immediately
(C) Encourage continued breastfeeding
(D) Delay feeding until symptoms resolve

Q614. A newborn presents with lethargy, poor feeding, and hypotonia within the first 24 hours of life, and laboratory findings confirm low calcium levels; what condition is most likely present?

(A) Neonatal hypoglycemia
(B) Neonatal infection process
(C) Neonatal hypocalcemia state
(D) Respiratory distress syndrome

Q615. A postpartum patient is being educated about signs of complications before discharge; which symptom should be reported immediately?

(A) Heavy vaginal bleeding
(B) Occasional mood changes
(C) Mild fatigue feeling
(D) Breast fullness sensation

Q616. A newborn develops rapid breathing, nasal flaring, and intercostal retractions shortly after birth; what is the most likely condition?
(A) Feeding difficulty
(B) Thermoregulation issue
(C) Normal transition process
(D) Respiratory distress condition
Q617. A postpartum patient asks about contraception options while breastfeeding and expresses concern about milk supply; which method is most appropriate?
(A) Progestin-only method
(B) Combined oral pills
(C) Estrogen therapy
(D) No contraception needed
Q618. A nurse observes a colleague documenting care that was not actually performed on a postpartum patient; what is the most appropriate action based on professional standards?
(A) Confront aggressively
(B) Report according to policy
(C) Ignore the situation
(D) Document similarly
Q619. A newborn requires stimulation at birth, has weak tone, and irregular respirations, but improves quickly with warming and suctioning; what does this indicate about neonatal adaptation?
(A) Circulatory collapse
(B) Mild transitional difficulty
(C) Neurological damage
(D) Severe respiratory failure
Q620. A postpartum patient is preparing for discharge and expresses concern about recognizing newborn illness, managing feeding schedules, and balancing self-care, while also reporting limited family support and anxiety about returning home; the nurse assesses readiness and identifies knowledge gaps. What is the most appropriate nursing action in this situation?
(A) Avoid discussing concerns
(B) Provide comprehensive discharge teaching
(C) Refer without education
(D) Delay discharge indefinitely
Q621. The primary hormone responsible for milk production during lactation is what?
(A) Prolactin hormone secretion
(B) Progesterone hormone action
(C) Estrogen hormone activity
(D) Oxytocin hormone release
Q622. A newborn with low blood glucose may exhibit which early clinical sign?
(A) Jitteriness and irritability
(B) Strong coordinated suck
(C) Pink skin coloration
(D) Regular sleep pattern
Q623. A postpartum patient reports severe breast pain, localized redness, fever, and chills while breastfeeding, and states that feeding has become increasingly difficult due to discomfort; what is the most appropriate nursing intervention?
(A) Encourage continued breastfeeding
(B) Switch to formula feeding
(C) Stop breastfeeding temporarily

(D) Decrease feeding frequency

Q624. A newborn demonstrates lethargy, weak cry, and poor feeding within the first day of life, and laboratory findings confirm elevated bilirubin levels; what condition is most likely present?

(A) Neonatal infection process
(B) Neonatal hypoglycemia
(C) Neonatal jaundice state
(D) Respiratory distress syndrome

Q625. A postpartum patient is instructed on warning signs before discharge; which symptom requires immediate reporting to a healthcare provider?

(A) Occasional mood changes
(B) Sudden severe headache
(C) Breast fullness sensation
(D) Mild fatigue feeling

Q626. A newborn develops grunting, nasal flaring, and chest retractions shortly after birth; what condition is most likely present?

(A) Normal adaptation process
(B) Respiratory distress condition
(C) Feeding difficulty issue
(D) Thermoregulation imbalance

Q627. A postpartum patient plans to return to work and asks how to maintain milk supply while separated from the infant; what is the most appropriate recommendation?

(A) Pump milk regularly
(B) Stop breastfeeding early
(C) Reduce feeding frequency
(D) Avoid milk expression

Q628. A nurse witnesses a breach of patient confidentiality when another staff member discusses patient information in a public area; what is the most appropriate action?

(A) Document similar actions
(B) Report the incident appropriately
(C) Join the conversation
(D) Ignore the behavior

Q629. A newborn shows delayed crying at birth, decreased tone, and irregular respirations but responds quickly to stimulation and warming; what does this indicate about neonatal adaptation?

(A) Severe respiratory failure
(B) Neurological impairment
(C) Mild transitional difficulty
(D) Circulatory collapse

Q630. A postpartum patient preparing for discharge expresses concern about breastfeeding challenges, newborn care, lack of support at home, and anxiety about recognizing complications, while demonstrating limited understanding of warning signs; the nurse performs a comprehensive assessment of needs and readiness. What is the most appropriate nursing action in this situation?

(A) Avoid addressing concerns
(B) Provide detailed education and resources
(C) Refer without explanation
(D) Delay discharge without planning

Q631. The primary antibody found in breast milk that provides neonatal immunity is what?

(A) Immunoglobulin M type
(B) Immunoglobulin G type

(C) Immunoglobulin E type
(D) Immunoglobulin A type
Q632. A newborn with hypoglycemia may also demonstrate which additional symptom besides jitteriness?
(A) Stable temperature
(B) Strong muscle tone
(C) Vigorous crying
(D) Poor feeding pattern
Q633. A postpartum patient reports persistent breast pain, fever, and redness, and states that breastfeeding is very painful but continues to feed the infant irregularly due to discomfort; what is the most appropriate nursing intervention?
(A) Stop breastfeeding immediately
(B) Reduce feeding frequency
(C) Switch completely to formula
(D) Encourage regular effective breastfeeding
Q634. A newborn develops yellow discoloration of the skin and sclera within the first 48 hours of life and shows mild lethargy; what condition is most likely present?
(A) Neonatal hypoglycemia
(B) Respiratory distress syndrome
(C) Neonatal jaundice state
(D) Neonatal infection process
Q635. A postpartum patient is taught discharge instructions; which symptom requires urgent medical evaluation?
(A) Occasional mood swings
(B) Mild fatigue feeling
(C) Breast fullness sensation
(D) Sudden chest pain onset
Q636. A newborn exhibits rapid breathing, grunting, and nasal flaring shortly after birth, along with decreased oxygen saturation; what condition is most likely present?
(A) Normal adaptation process
(B) Thermoregulation imbalance
(C) Feeding difficulty issue
(D) Respiratory distress condition
Q637. A postpartum patient returning to work asks how to store expressed breast milk safely while maintaining quality; what is the most appropriate recommendation?
(A) Leave milk at room temperature
(B) Avoid refrigeration completely
(C) Discard milk after pumping
(D) Store milk in clean containers
Q638. A nurse identifies that a colleague administered medication without verifying patient identity, violating safety protocols; what is the most appropriate action?
(A) Confront without reporting
(B) Report according to safety policy
(C) Ignore the situation
(D) Document similarly
Q639. A newborn demonstrates weak cry, decreased tone, and slow respiratory effort immediately after birth but responds well to stimulation and warming within a few minutes; what does this indicate about neonatal adaptation?

(A) Neurological impairment
(B) Circulatory collapse
(C) Severe respiratory failure
(D) Mild transitional difficulty

Q640. A postpartum patient preparing for discharge expresses concerns about breastfeeding difficulties, newborn illness recognition, safe sleep practices, and lack of family support, while also demonstrating limited understanding of warning signs and anxiety about managing care independently; the nurse completes a comprehensive assessment of readiness. What is the most appropriate nursing action in this situation?
(A) Avoid discussing patient concerns
(B) Provide individualized discharge education and resources
(C) Delay discharge without explanation
(D) Refer without providing guidance

Q641. The hormone responsible for uterine contractions during breastfeeding is what?
(A) Progesterone hormone action
(B) Oxytocin hormone release
(C) Prolactin hormone secretion
(D) Estrogen hormone activity

Q642. A newborn experiencing hypothermia may exhibit which early sign?
(A) Cold skin temperature
(B) Strong feeding pattern
(C) Increased activity level
(D) Elevated body warmth

Q643. A postpartum patient reports that breasts feel extremely full, tight, and painful, especially before feeding, but symptoms improve significantly after breastfeeding; what is the most appropriate nursing intervention?
(A) Switch to formula feeding
(B) Reduce feeding frequency
(C) Stop breastfeeding temporarily
(D) Encourage frequent feeding

Q644. A newborn presents with poor feeding, lethargy, and low blood glucose levels shortly after birth; what condition is most likely present?
(A) Neonatal infection process
(B) Respiratory distress syndrome
(C) Neonatal hypoglycemia state
(D) Neonatal jaundice condition

Q645. A postpartum patient is educated on warning signs of thromboembolism; which symptom requires immediate reporting?
(A) Breast fullness sensation
(B) Mild fatigue feeling
(C) Unilateral leg pain
(D) Occasional mood swings

Q646. A newborn develops nasal flaring, grunting, and intercostal retractions shortly after birth, with decreased oxygen saturation levels; what condition is most likely present?
(A) Respiratory distress condition
(B) Thermoregulation imbalance
(C) Normal transition process
(D) Feeding difficulty issue

Q647. A postpartum patient returning to work asks how to maintain milk supply during long work hours and separation from the infant; what is the most appropriate recommendation?
(A) Avoid milk expression
(B) Reduce feeding frequency
(C) Stop breastfeeding early
(D) Pump at regular intervals
Q648. A nurse observes a medication error made by a colleague but no harm has occurred to the patient; what is the most appropriate action based on safety principles?
(A) Ignore since no harm
(B) Confront without reporting
(C) Document similar behavior
(D) Report the error promptly
Q649. A newborn demonstrates weak cry, decreased tone, and irregular respirations immediately after birth but responds rapidly to stimulation and warming; what does this indicate about neonatal adaptation?
(A) Neurological impairment
(B) Severe respiratory failure
(C) Circulatory collapse
(D) Mild transitional difficulty
Q650. A postpartum patient preparing for discharge expresses concerns about breastfeeding challenges, safe sleep practices, recognizing newborn illness, and limited social support, while also demonstrating anxiety and incomplete understanding of care instructions; the nurse conducts a full readiness assessment. What is the most appropriate nursing action in this situation?
(A) Refer without education
(B) Provide individualized teaching and support
(C) Avoid addressing concerns
(D) Delay discharge indefinitely
Q651. The reflex responsible for coordinating sucking, swallowing, and breathing in a newborn is what?
(A) Feeding coordination reflex
(B) Tonic neck reflex
(C) Moro reflex response
(D) Babinski reflex action
Q652. A newborn exposed to cold stress may develop which metabolic complication?
(A) Hyperglycemia condition
(B) Hypoglycemia condition
(C) Increased oxygen level
(D) Elevated calcium level
Q653. A postpartum patient reports that breasts feel hard, swollen, and painful before feeding, and notes that symptoms improve after breastfeeding sessions, especially when feeding occurs more frequently; what is the most appropriate nursing intervention?
(A) Switch to formula feeding
(B) Encourage frequent breastfeeding
(C) Reduce feeding frequency
(D) Stop breastfeeding temporarily
Q654. A newborn develops tremors, high-pitched cry, and irritability within hours of birth, and laboratory findings indicate low blood glucose levels; what condition is most likely present?
(A) Neonatal hypoglycemia state

(B) Respiratory distress syndrome
(C) Neonatal jaundice condition
(D) Neonatal infection process

Q655. A postpartum patient is instructed on signs of infection before discharge; which symptom should be reported immediately?
(A) Breast fullness sensation
(B) Occasional mood swings
(C) Foul-smelling vaginal discharge
(D) Mild fatigue feeling

Q656. A newborn presents with grunting, nasal flaring, retractions, and decreased oxygen saturation levels shortly after birth; what is the most likely condition?
(A) Normal transition process
(B) Feeding difficulty issue
(C) Thermoregulation imbalance
(D) Respiratory distress condition

Q657. A postpartum patient plans to exclusively pump breast milk due to work constraints and asks how to maintain adequate supply; what is the most appropriate recommendation?
(A) Avoid nighttime pumping
(B) Stop milk expression early
(C) Reduce pumping frequency
(D) Pump at consistent intervals

Q658. A nurse observes a breach in sterile technique during a postpartum procedure by a colleague; what is the most appropriate action?
(A) Ignore the observation
(B) Confront without reporting
(C) Report according to protocol
(D) Document similar actions

Q659. A newborn demonstrates delayed crying, decreased tone, and irregular respirations immediately after birth but responds quickly to stimulation and warming within a few minutes; what does this indicate about neonatal adaptation?
(A) Neurological impairment
(B) Mild transitional difficulty
(C) Circulatory collapse
(D) Severe respiratory failure

Q660. A postpartum patient preparing for discharge reports concerns about breastfeeding challenges, recognizing newborn complications, maintaining safe sleep practices, and managing care independently due to limited support at home, while demonstrating anxiety and incomplete understanding of instructions; the nurse completes a comprehensive readiness assessment. What is the most appropriate nursing action in this situation?
(A) Delay discharge without explanation
(B) Avoid addressing concerns
(C) Refer without providing guidance
(D) Provide tailored education and support resources

Q661. The component in breast milk that provides protection against gastrointestinal infections is what?
(A) Secretory immunoglobulin A
(B) Mineral electrolyte level
(C) Lactose carbohydrate content

(D) Fatty acid concentration

Q662. A newborn experiencing hypoglycemia may also show which neurological sign?

(A) Strong muscle tone
(B) Coordinated movement
(C) Quiet sleep pattern
(D) Tremors or jitteriness

Q663. A postpartum patient reports breast engorgement with swelling, firmness, and discomfort that improves after feeding, and asks how to prevent recurrence during the next few days; what is the most appropriate nursing intervention?

(A) Decrease feeding frequency
(B) Encourage frequent and regular feeding
(C) Stop breastfeeding temporarily
(D) Replace feeding with formula

Q664. A newborn develops yellow discoloration of the skin within 24-48 hours, along with mild lethargy and decreased feeding interest; what condition is most likely present?

(A) Respiratory distress syndrome
(B) Neonatal infection process
(C) Neonatal jaundice state
(D) Neonatal hypoglycemia

Q665. A postpartum patient is instructed on signs of thromboembolism; which symptom should be reported immediately?

(A) Sudden shortness of breath
(B) Breast fullness sensation
(C) Mild fatigue feeling
(D) Occasional mood swings

Q666. A newborn presents with grunting, nasal flaring, retractions, and decreased oxygen saturation shortly after birth, requiring supplemental oxygen; what condition is most likely present?

(A) Normal transition process
(B) Thermoregulation imbalance
(C) Feeding difficulty issue
(D) Respiratory distress condition

Q667. A postpartum patient asks how to safely store expressed breast milk at home while maintaining its quality and safety for the newborn over several days; what is the most appropriate recommendation?

(A) Leave milk at room temperature
(B) Avoid refrigeration completely
(C) Store milk in sterile containers
(D) Discard milk immediately

Q668. A nurse observes another staff member discussing patient information loudly in a public hallway where visitors are present; what is the most appropriate professional action?

(A) Document similar actions
(B) Participate in discussion
(C) Report breach of confidentiality
(D) Ignore the behavior

Q669. A newborn demonstrates weak cry, decreased tone, and irregular respirations at birth but shows rapid improvement after stimulation, warming, and minimal suctioning; what does this indicate about neonatal adaptation?

(A) Severe respiratory failure

(B) Neurological impairment
(C) Circulatory collapse
(D) Mild transitional difficulty

Q670. A postpartum patient preparing for discharge expresses concerns about breastfeeding effectiveness, recognizing newborn complications, safe sleep positioning, and managing care independently due to limited support, while also demonstrating anxiety and incomplete understanding of instructions despite prior teaching; the nurse reassesses readiness and identifies multiple learning needs. What is the most appropriate nursing action in this situation?
(A) Delay discharge without explanation
(B) Avoid addressing concerns
(C) Refer without additional education
(D) Provide individualized teaching with reinforcement

Q671. The primary benefit of early breastfeeding within the first hour after birth is what?
(A) Delays infant feeding
(B) Reduces maternal fatigue
(C) Stimulates milk production
(D) Prevents infant crying

Q672. A newborn experiencing hypocalcemia may exhibit which symptom?
(A) Stable body temperature
(B) Muscle twitching or jitteriness
(C) Strong feeding pattern
(D) Calm behavior state

Q673. A postpartum patient reports that breastfeeding sessions are irregular due to pain, leading to increased breast fullness and discomfort between feeds, and asks how to manage symptoms effectively; what is the most appropriate nursing intervention?
(A) Switch to formula feeding
(B) Encourage consistent feeding schedule
(C) Decrease feeding frequency
(D) Stop breastfeeding temporarily

Q674. A newborn develops yellow discoloration of the skin and sclera within the first 2 days of life and shows mild lethargy with decreased feeding interest; what condition is most likely present?
(A) Respiratory distress syndrome
(B) Neonatal infection process
(C) Neonatal hypoglycemia
(D) Neonatal jaundice state

Q675. A postpartum patient is educated about warning signs of infection before discharge; which symptom requires immediate reporting?
(A) Mild fatigue feeling
(B) Fever above normal range
(C) Occasional mood swings
(D) Breast fullness sensation

Q676. A newborn presents with nasal flaring, grunting, retractions, and decreased oxygen saturation shortly after birth, requiring respiratory support; what condition is most likely present?
(A) Thermoregulation imbalance
(B) Respiratory distress condition
(C) Feeding difficulty issue
(D) Normal transition process

Q677. A postpartum patient plans to store expressed breast milk and asks how long it can be safely kept in a refrigerator while maintaining its nutritional quality; what is the most appropriate recommendation?
(A) Avoid refrigeration completely
(B) Discard milk immediately
(C) Leave milk at room temperature
(D) Follow safe refrigeration guidelines
Q678. A nurse observes a colleague failing to perform hand hygiene before providing care to a postpartum patient; what is the most appropriate action?
(A) Ignore the behavior
(B) Confront without reporting
(C) Report according to infection control policy
(D) Document similar behavior
Q679. A newborn demonstrates weak cry, decreased tone, and irregular respirations immediately after birth but responds rapidly to stimulation, warming, and minimal airway clearing; what does this indicate about neonatal adaptation?
(A) Severe respiratory failure
(B) Circulatory collapse
(C) Neurological impairment
(D) Mild transitional difficulty
Q680. A postpartum patient preparing for discharge reports concerns about breastfeeding effectiveness, recognizing newborn complications, safe sleep positioning, and managing care independently due to limited support, while also demonstrating anxiety and incomplete understanding despite prior teaching sessions; the nurse reassesses readiness and identifies ongoing learning needs. What is the most appropriate nursing action in this situation?
(A) Refer without further teaching
(B) Delay discharge without explanation
(C) Avoid addressing concerns
(D) Provide repeated individualized education
Q681. The hormone that maintains milk production through regular breastfeeding stimulation is what?
(A) Prolactin hormone secretion
(B) Oxytocin hormone release
(C) Estrogen hormone activity
(D) Progesterone hormone action
Q682. A newborn with hypothermia may also develop which metabolic disturbance due to increased energy use?
(A) Elevated calcium level
(B) Hypoglycemia condition
(C) Increased sodium level
(D) Hyperglycemia condition
Q683. A postpartum patient reports nipple pain and cracking during breastfeeding, and states that the infant frequently loses latch and feeds for prolonged periods without satisfaction; what is the most appropriate nursing intervention?
(A) Switch completely to formula
(B) Assess and correct latch technique
(C) Stop breastfeeding temporarily
(D) Decrease feeding frequency

Q684. A newborn presents with tremors, irritability, and poor feeding within the first hours of life, and blood glucose testing confirms low levels; what condition is most likely present?
(A) Neonatal infection process
(B) Neonatal jaundice condition
(C) Respiratory distress syndrome
(D) Neonatal hypoglycemia state
Q685. A postpartum patient is educated on warning signs before discharge; which symptom should be reported immediately to prevent serious complications?
(A) Occasional mood swings
(B) Mild fatigue feeling
(C) Breast fullness sensation
(D) Sudden visual disturbances
Q686. A newborn develops grunting, nasal flaring, and chest retractions shortly after birth, along with decreasing oxygen saturation levels requiring support; what condition is most likely present?
(A) Normal transition process
(B) Respiratory distress condition
(C) Feeding difficulty issue
(D) Thermoregulation imbalance
Q687. A postpartum patient asks how to maintain milk supply while exclusively pumping due to infant separation and work commitments, and expresses concern about decreased production over time; what is the most appropriate recommendation?
(A) Stop pumping during night
(B) Avoid frequent milk expression
(C) Pump at consistent frequent intervals
(D) Reduce pumping sessions gradually
Q688. A nurse notices a colleague bypassing safety checks when administering medications to a postpartum patient, increasing the risk of error; what is the most appropriate professional action?
(A) Document similar practice
(B) Ignore the behavior
(C) Confront without reporting
(D) Report according to safety policy
Q689. A newborn demonstrates weak cry, decreased tone, and irregular respirations immediately after birth but responds quickly to stimulation, warming, and airway clearing within a few minutes; what does this indicate about neonatal adaptation?
(A) Mild transitional difficulty
(B) Neurological impairment
(C) Severe respiratory failure
(D) Circulatory collapse
Q690. A postpartum patient preparing for discharge expresses multiple concerns about breastfeeding effectiveness, recognizing newborn complications, safe sleep practices, and managing care independently due to lack of support, while also showing anxiety and incomplete understanding despite repeated teaching sessions; the nurse reassesses readiness and identifies persistent learning gaps. What is the most appropriate nursing action in this situation?
(A) Avoid addressing ongoing concerns
(B) Delay discharge without explanation
(C) Refer without additional teaching
(D) Provide repeated individualized education and support
Q691. The initial milk produced in the first few days after birth is known as what?

(A) Stored gland milk
(B) Mature breast milk
(C) Transitional stage milk
(D) Colostrum early milk

Q692. A newborn with hypocalcemia may also present with which additional neurological sign?
(A) Calm sleep pattern
(B) Strong coordinated movement
(C) Stable feeding ability
(D) Seizure-like activity

Q693. A postpartum patient reports persistent nipple soreness with visible cracks and states the infant feeds frequently but seems unsatisfied after each session; what is the most appropriate nursing intervention?
(A) Reduce feeding frequency
(B) Reassess latch and positioning technique
(C) Switch fully to formula
(D) Stop breastfeeding temporarily

Q694. A newborn demonstrates lethargy, weak cry, and poor feeding within hours after birth, and blood glucose testing confirms significantly low levels; what condition is most likely present?
(A) Neonatal hypoglycemia state
(B) Neonatal jaundice condition
(C) Respiratory distress syndrome
(D) Neonatal infection process

Q695. A postpartum patient is educated on signs of postpartum complications; which symptom requires immediate evaluation?
(A) Mild fatigue feeling
(B) Occasional mood changes
(C) Breast fullness sensation
(D) Sudden severe abdominal pain

Q696. A newborn exhibits persistent tachypnea, nasal flaring, and chest retractions, along with low oxygen saturation despite initial support measures; what condition is most likely present?
(A) Thermoregulation imbalance
(B) Normal transition process
(C) Respiratory distress condition
(D) Feeding difficulty issue

Q697. A postpartum patient who is exclusively pumping reports decreasing milk output over the past few days and states that pumping sessions have become irregular due to fatigue and schedule changes; what is the most appropriate nursing recommendation?
(A) Decrease pumping frequency
(B) Stop pumping temporarily
(C) Avoid nighttime sessions
(D) Reinforce consistent pumping schedule

Q698. A nurse observes a colleague failing to verify patient identification before administering medication to a postpartum patient, increasing the risk of error; what is the most appropriate professional response?
(A) Report according to institutional policy
(B) Ignore since no harm occurred
(C) Document similar behavior
(D) Confront without escalation

Q699. A newborn presents with weak respiratory effort, decreased muscle tone, and delayed crying immediately after birth but demonstrates rapid improvement following stimulation, warming, and airway clearing within a few minutes; what does this indicate about neonatal transition?
(A) Circulatory collapse
(B) Neurological impairment
(C) Mild transitional difficulty
(D) Severe respiratory failure
Q700. A postpartum patient preparing for discharge reports ongoing concerns about breastfeeding success, newborn illness recognition, safe sleep practices, and independent care due to minimal support at home, while also demonstrating anxiety and repeated misunderstanding of key instructions despite prior teaching; the nurse reassesses readiness and identifies persistent educational gaps. What is the most appropriate nursing action in this situation?
(A) Avoid further discussion of concerns
(B) Refer without additional guidance
(C) Provide repeated structured education with reinforcement
(D) Delay discharge without explanation

Answer Key and Explanation (601-700)

Q601. Answer: A

Explanation: The milk ejection reflex is controlled by oxytocin released from the posterior pituitary. This hormone causes contraction of the milk ducts, allowing milk to flow toward the nipple. It is triggered by infant suckling and emotional cues. Prolactin is responsible for milk production, not ejection. Effective let-down is essential for successful breastfeeding. This mechanism supports neonatal nutrition and bonding. ##

Q602. Answer: A

Explanation: Frequent feeding on demand is recommended during the early postpartum period. This helps establish milk supply and prevents engorgement. Newborns typically feed every 2-3 hours. Responding to feeding cues supports adequate nutrition. It also promotes bonding between mother and infant. Consistent feeding patterns improve lactation success. ##

Q603. Answer: D

Explanation: Cracked nipples and pain are often caused by improper latch. Evaluating positioning ensures the infant takes in adequate breast tissue. Correct latch reduces friction and prevents further injury. Continued breastfeeding with proper technique promotes healing. Education and support improve breastfeeding success. Early intervention prevents complications. ##

Q604. Answer: A

Explanation: Jitteriness and poor feeding are common signs of neonatal hypoglycemia. Low blood glucose levels affect neurological function. Early detection is essential to prevent complications. Feeding or glucose administration helps restore levels. Monitoring ensures stabilization. This condition is more common in certain high-risk infants. ##

Q605. Answer: C

Explanation: Positive pressure ventilation is the first step when a newborn fails to breathe effectively. Adequate ventilation improves oxygenation and heart rate. Chest compressions are initiated only if heart rate remains low after ventilation. Early intervention is critical for survival. Monitoring response guides further actions. Timely care improves neonatal outcomes. ##

Q606. Answer: D

Explanation: Postpartum blues are common in the early days after delivery. Symptoms include mood swings, tearfulness, and emotional sensitivity. These changes are related to hormonal shifts. They typically resolve within two weeks. Support and reassurance are important. Monitoring ensures symptoms do not worsen. ##

Q607. Answer: A

Explanation: Hypothermia occurs when a newborn loses heat faster than it can produce it. This can lead to metabolic complications. Maintaining warmth is essential for stability. Interventions include skin-to-skin contact and warming devices. Monitoring temperature ensures effectiveness. Early management prevents further complications. ##

Q608. Answer: A

Explanation: Unilateral swelling and pain suggest deep vein thrombosis. Pregnancy and postpartum increase clotting risk. Early recognition is critical to prevent complications. Treatment typically involves anticoagulation. Monitoring ensures prevention of embolism. This condition requires prompt medical attention. ##

Q609. Answer: A

Explanation: Mild difficulty in adaptation may require minimal stimulation. Improvement with intervention suggests adequate recovery ability. Weak cry and tone initially indicate slight delay. Monitoring ensures continued progress. Most infants stabilize quickly. This reflects a transient adjustment issue. ##

Q610. Answer: D
Explanation: Education helps address misconceptions about breastfeeding. Support resources can assist with work-related concerns. Providing options empowers informed decision-making. Emotional support improves confidence. Continued guidance promotes successful feeding practices. This approach supports patient-centered care and outcomes. ##
Q611. Answer: B
Explanation: Colostrum is the first milk produced after delivery and is rich in antibodies. It provides essential immune protection to the newborn. The thick consistency supports concentrated nutrient delivery. It is produced in small amounts but is highly beneficial. This milk supports early gut immunity and development. It transitions into mature milk over time. ##
Q612. Answer: D
Explanation: When the heart rate remains below 60 despite adequate ventilation, chest compressions are indicated. Effective ventilation is always the first priority. Compressions help improve circulation and oxygen delivery. The combination of ventilation and compressions supports recovery. Continuous reassessment is required during resuscitation. Prompt intervention improves survival outcomes. ##
Q613. Answer: C
Explanation: Mastitis is characterized by breast pain, redness, and systemic symptoms. Continued breastfeeding helps empty the breast and reduce infection. It prevents worsening of milk stasis. Antibiotics may be required for treatment. Supportive care improves recovery. Early intervention prevents complications. ##
Q614. Answer: C
Explanation: Hypocalcemia in newborns can present with lethargy and poor feeding. Low calcium affects neuromuscular function. Early identification is important to prevent complications. Treatment includes calcium supplementation. Monitoring ensures normalization of levels. This condition requires prompt management. ##
Q615. Answer: A
Explanation: Heavy vaginal bleeding may indicate postpartum hemorrhage. It requires immediate medical evaluation. Early recognition prevents severe complications. Patients should be educated on warning signs. Monitoring bleeding patterns is essential. Prompt reporting ensures timely intervention. ##
Q616. Answer: D
Explanation: Rapid breathing and retractions are signs of respiratory distress. These symptoms indicate difficulty maintaining adequate oxygenation. Early intervention is required to support breathing. Monitoring oxygen levels is essential. Treatment depends on severity. Prompt care improves neonatal outcomes. ##
Q617. Answer: A
Explanation: Progestin-only methods are preferred during breastfeeding. They do not interfere with milk production. Estrogen-containing methods may reduce supply. Early contraception planning prevents unintended pregnancy. Education supports informed choices. This method is safe and effective postpartum. ##
Q618. Answer: B
Explanation: Falsifying documentation is a serious ethical violation. Reporting ensures patient safety and accountability. Following institutional policy maintains professionalism. Ignoring the issue can harm patients. Ethical practice is essential in healthcare. This action supports legal and professional standards. ##
Q619. Answer: B
Explanation: Some newborns require minimal assistance during transition. Improvement with simple interventions indicates mild difficulty. This is common and usually resolves quickly. Monitoring ensures

continued stability. No advanced intervention is needed if recovery occurs. This reflects a transient adjustment process. ##

Q620. Answer: B

Explanation: Comprehensive discharge teaching addresses patient concerns and knowledge gaps. Education improves confidence in newborn care. Providing clear instructions supports safe transition home. Emotional support helps reduce anxiety. Resources can assist with limited support systems. This approach promotes patient safety and independence. ##

Q621. Answer: A

Explanation: Prolactin is the hormone responsible for stimulating milk production in the mammary glands. It is released from the anterior pituitary gland in response to infant suckling. Higher levels of prolactin support increased milk synthesis. This process is essential for maintaining an adequate milk supply. Oxytocin, in contrast, is responsible for milk ejection. Effective lactation depends on proper hormonal balance. ##

Q622. Answer: A

Explanation: Jitteriness is one of the earliest signs of neonatal hypoglycemia. Low glucose levels affect neurological stability. Irritability may also be present due to decreased energy supply. Early detection is critical to prevent complications. Feeding or glucose administration helps correct the imbalance. Monitoring ensures stabilization of glucose levels. ##

Q623. Answer: A

Explanation: Mastitis is characterized by pain, redness, and systemic symptoms. Continued breastfeeding helps empty the breast and reduce milk stasis. This prevents worsening of infection and promotes healing. Antibiotics may be required for treatment. Supportive care improves comfort and recovery. Early management reduces complications. ##

Q624. Answer: C

Explanation: Elevated bilirubin levels lead to neonatal jaundice. Symptoms may include lethargy and poor feeding. Early recognition is important to prevent complications. Treatment may involve phototherapy. Monitoring bilirubin levels guides management. This condition is common in newborns. ##

Q625. Answer: B

Explanation: A sudden severe headache may indicate serious complications such as hypertension or neurological issues. Early recognition is essential for timely intervention. This symptom should not be ignored. Patients should be educated on danger signs before discharge. Prompt reporting improves outcomes. Monitoring ensures patient safety. ##

Q626. Answer: B

Explanation: Grunting and retractions are signs of respiratory distress. These symptoms indicate difficulty maintaining adequate oxygenation. Early intervention is required to support breathing. Monitoring oxygen saturation is essential. Treatment depends on severity. Prompt care improves neonatal outcomes. ##

Q627. Answer: A

Explanation: Regular pumping helps maintain milk supply when separated from the infant. It mimics the natural feeding pattern and stimulates prolactin release. Consistency is key to preventing decreased production. Stored milk can be used for feeding later. Education supports continued breastfeeding success. This approach helps balance work and lactation. ##

Q628. Answer: B

Explanation: Maintaining patient confidentiality is a legal and ethical responsibility. Discussing patient information in public areas violates privacy standards. Reporting ensures accountability and prevention of future incidents. Following institutional policy is essential. Protecting patient information maintains trust. This action supports professional integrity. ##

Q629. Answer: C
Explanation: Some newborns require minimal assistance during transition. Improvement with simple interventions indicates mild difficulty. Delayed crying and tone initially suggest slight delay. Rapid response shows adequate recovery ability. Monitoring ensures stability continues. This reflects a temporary adaptation issue. ##
Q630. Answer: B
Explanation: Providing education addresses knowledge gaps and improves confidence. Resources help support the patient after discharge. Clear instructions ensure recognition of warning signs. Emotional support reduces anxiety and promotes readiness. Patient-centered care improves outcomes. This approach ensures safe transition to home. ##
Q631. Answer: D
Explanation: Immunoglobulin A is the main antibody present in breast milk. It provides passive immunity by protecting mucosal surfaces. This antibody helps prevent infections in the newborn. It is especially important for gastrointestinal protection. Breastfeeding enhances immune defense during early life. This supports overall neonatal health and development. ##
Q632. Answer: D
Explanation: Poor feeding is a common symptom of neonatal hypoglycemia. Low glucose levels reduce energy availability. This affects feeding ability and overall activity. Early recognition is important to prevent complications. Treatment includes feeding or glucose administration. Monitoring ensures stabilization of glucose levels. ##
Q633. Answer: D
Explanation: Mastitis requires continued breast emptying to prevent worsening. Irregular feeding can lead to milk stasis and increased infection. Encouraging regular feeding helps clear blocked ducts. Proper technique reduces discomfort and promotes healing. Antibiotics may be needed depending on severity. Early intervention improves recovery outcomes. ##
Q634. Answer: C
Explanation: Yellow discoloration of the skin indicates elevated bilirubin levels. This condition is known as neonatal jaundice. Mild lethargy can occur as bilirubin rises. Early assessment is important to determine severity. Treatment may involve phototherapy. Monitoring prevents complications such as bilirubin toxicity. ##
Q635. Answer: D
Explanation: Sudden chest pain may indicate a serious condition such as pulmonary embolism. Postpartum patients are at increased risk for thromboembolic events. Immediate evaluation is necessary. Early recognition can prevent life-threatening complications. Education helps patients identify warning signs. Prompt reporting ensures timely care. ##
Q636. Answer: D
Explanation: These signs indicate difficulty with oxygenation and ventilation. Respiratory distress requires immediate assessment and support. Decreased oxygen saturation confirms inadequate gas exchange. Early intervention improves outcomes. Monitoring ensures stabilization. Treatment depends on severity and cause. ##
Q637. Answer: D
Explanation: Proper storage of breast milk is essential to maintain safety and quality. Clean containers prevent contamination. Refrigeration or freezing preserves nutrients and prevents bacterial growth. Guidelines should be followed for storage duration. Education supports safe feeding practices. This helps maintain infant health. ##
Q638. Answer: B
Explanation: Patient safety requires strict adherence to identification protocols. Violations can lead to serious harm. Reporting ensures accountability and prevention of future errors. Following institutional

policy supports safe practice. Ignoring the issue compromises patient care. This action promotes a culture of safety. ##

Q639. Answer: D

Explanation: Some newborns require minimal support during transition. Improvement with stimulation indicates mild adaptation delay. Weak initial responses are not uncommon. Rapid recovery suggests adequate physiological reserves. Monitoring ensures continued stability. This reflects a temporary adjustment process. ##

Q640. Answer: B

Explanation: Individualized education addresses specific patient concerns and knowledge gaps. Providing resources supports care after discharge. Clear guidance improves confidence and safety. Addressing emotional concerns reduces anxiety. Patient-centered teaching promotes independence. This approach ensures a safe transition to home care. ##

Q641. Answer: B

Explanation: Oxytocin is released during breastfeeding and causes uterine contractions. These contractions help reduce uterine size after delivery. They also assist in preventing excessive bleeding. The hormone is triggered by infant suckling. This mechanism supports postpartum recovery. It works alongside prolactin, which produces milk. ##

Q642. Answer: A

Explanation: Hypothermia occurs when a newborn loses heat rapidly. Cold skin is one of the earliest signs. It can lead to metabolic stress if not corrected. Maintaining warmth is essential for stability. Early intervention prevents complications. Monitoring ensures temperature normalization. ##

Q643. Answer: D

Explanation: Breast engorgement occurs due to accumulation of milk. Frequent feeding helps empty the breasts and relieve discomfort. This prevents worsening of symptoms. Proper latch and positioning should also be reinforced. Monitoring ensures improvement. This approach supports continued breastfeeding success. ##

Q644. Answer: C

Explanation: Hypoglycemia affects energy supply to the newborn. Symptoms include lethargy and poor feeding. Early detection is critical to prevent neurological damage. Treatment includes feeding or glucose administration. Monitoring ensures stabilization of glucose levels. This condition is common in high-risk infants. ##

Q645. Answer: C

Explanation: Unilateral leg pain may indicate deep vein thrombosis. Postpartum patients are at increased risk for clot formation. Early recognition is essential to prevent embolism. Patients should be educated on warning signs. Prompt reporting ensures timely treatment. This improves patient safety outcomes. ##

Q646. Answer: A

Explanation: These symptoms indicate impaired respiratory function. Grunting and retractions show increased work of breathing. Decreased oxygen saturation confirms inadequate oxygenation. Immediate intervention is necessary. Monitoring supports evaluation of response. Early treatment improves neonatal outcomes. ##

Q647. Answer: D

Explanation: Regular pumping mimics infant feeding patterns. This helps maintain prolactin levels and milk production. Consistency is essential for supply maintenance. Expressed milk can be stored for later use. Education supports continued breastfeeding success. This approach helps balance work and lactation. ##

Q648. Answer: D

Explanation: Reporting errors is essential even if no harm occurs. It helps identify system issues and prevent future errors. Transparency supports patient safety culture. Following institutional policy is required. Ignoring errors can lead to repeated mistakes. This action promotes quality improvement. ##

Q649. Answer: D

Explanation: Some newborns require minimal support during transition. Rapid improvement indicates mild difficulty. Weak initial responses can occur during adaptation. Recovery with simple measures shows adequate physiological reserve. Monitoring ensures continued stability. This reflects a temporary adjustment process. ##

Q650. Answer: B

Explanation: Individualized teaching addresses specific concerns and knowledge gaps. Providing support improves confidence in caregiving. Education ensures understanding of warning signs. Addressing anxiety promotes readiness for discharge. Resources help compensate for limited support. This approach ensures safe transition to home care. ##

Q651. Answer: A

Explanation: The feeding coordination reflex allows newborns to suck, swallow, and breathe effectively. This coordination is essential for safe feeding. It ensures that the infant receives adequate nutrition without aspiration. The reflex develops during gestation and is present at birth. Assessment of this reflex helps evaluate neurological function. Proper coordination supports healthy growth and development. ##

Q652. Answer: B

Explanation: Cold stress increases metabolic demand in newborns. This leads to increased glucose consumption. As a result, hypoglycemia may develop. Maintaining warmth helps prevent this complication. Early detection is important for management. Monitoring ensures stabilization of metabolic status. ##

Q653. Answer: B

Explanation: Breast engorgement occurs when milk accumulates in the breast tissue. Frequent breastfeeding helps relieve pressure and discomfort. This prevents worsening of symptoms and promotes milk flow. Proper latch and positioning should also be reinforced. Monitoring ensures improvement. Continued feeding supports successful lactation. ##

Q654. Answer: A

Explanation: Hypoglycemia can present with neurological symptoms such as tremors and irritability. A high-pitched cry is also a concerning sign. Low glucose levels affect brain function. Early recognition is critical to prevent complications. Treatment includes feeding or glucose administration. Monitoring ensures stabilization of glucose levels. ##

Q655. Answer: C

Explanation: Foul-smelling discharge may indicate infection of the reproductive tract. Early recognition is essential for treatment. Patients should be educated on warning signs. Prompt reporting allows timely intervention. Monitoring helps prevent complications. This supports safe postpartum recovery. ##

Q656. Answer: D

Explanation: These signs indicate difficulty with breathing and oxygenation. Respiratory distress requires immediate intervention. Decreased oxygen saturation confirms inadequate gas exchange. Monitoring is essential for management. Treatment depends on severity. Early intervention improves outcomes. ##

Q657. Answer: D

Explanation: Consistent pumping mimics infant feeding patterns. This helps maintain prolactin levels and milk production. Regular intervals are important for sustaining supply. Skipping sessions can decrease production. Education supports successful lactation management. This approach helps meet infant nutritional needs. ##

Q658. Answer: C

Explanation: Maintaining sterile technique is essential to prevent infection. Breaches in protocol can compromise patient safety. Reporting ensures accountability and correction of practice. Following institutional guidelines is necessary. Ignoring the issue may lead to complications. This action supports quality and safety standards. ##

Q659. Answer: B

Explanation: Some newborns require minimal assistance during transition. Rapid improvement indicates mild difficulty. Delayed initial responses are not uncommon. Recovery with simple measures shows adequate physiological reserve. Monitoring ensures continued stability. This reflects a temporary adaptation process. ##

Q660. Answer: D

Explanation: Tailored education addresses specific knowledge gaps and concerns. Providing resources supports the patient after discharge. Clear instructions improve confidence and safety. Addressing emotional concerns reduces anxiety. Patient-centered care promotes independence. This approach ensures a safe transition to home. ##

Q661. Answer: A

Explanation: Secretory immunoglobulin A is a key immune component of breast milk. It coats the infant's gastrointestinal tract and prevents pathogen attachment. This provides passive immunity during early life. It is especially important in preventing infections. Breastfeeding enhances neonatal immune protection. This supports overall infant health and development. ##

Q662. Answer: D

Explanation: Tremors are a common neurological sign of hypoglycemia. Low glucose affects brain function and stability. Jitteriness indicates early neurological involvement. Prompt recognition is important for treatment. Feeding or glucose administration corrects the condition. Monitoring ensures stabilization of blood glucose levels. ##

Q663. Answer: B

Explanation: Frequent feeding prevents accumulation of milk in the breasts. This reduces engorgement and discomfort. Regular emptying maintains milk flow and supply. Proper latch and positioning should also be reinforced. Monitoring ensures symptoms improve. This approach supports effective lactation management. ##

Q664. Answer: C

Explanation: Yellow discoloration indicates elevated bilirubin levels. This condition is known as neonatal jaundice. Mild lethargy and poor feeding may accompany it. Early assessment determines severity. Treatment may involve phototherapy. Monitoring prevents complications such as bilirubin toxicity. ##

Q665. Answer: A

Explanation: Sudden shortness of breath may indicate pulmonary embolism. Postpartum patients are at increased risk for clot formation. Early recognition is critical for survival. Immediate medical evaluation is required. Education helps patients identify warning signs. Prompt reporting ensures timely intervention. ##

Q666. Answer: D

Explanation: These signs indicate impaired respiratory function. Grunting and retractions reflect increased work of breathing. Low oxygen saturation confirms inadequate gas exchange. Immediate intervention is required. Monitoring guides treatment decisions. Early management improves neonatal outcomes. ##

Q667. Answer: C

Explanation: Proper storage in sterile containers prevents contamination. Refrigeration or freezing preserves milk quality. Following guidelines ensures safety for the infant. Clean handling techniques are essential. Education supports proper storage practices. This helps maintain nutritional and immunological benefits. ##

Q668. Answer: C
Explanation: Discussing patient information in public violates confidentiality. Protecting patient privacy is a legal and ethical responsibility. Reporting ensures accountability and prevention of future breaches. Following institutional policy is essential. Ignoring the issue compromises trust. This action supports professional standards and patient rights. ##
Q669. Answer: D
Explanation: Some newborns require minimal support during transition. Rapid improvement indicates mild adaptation difficulty. Weak initial responses are not uncommon. Recovery with simple interventions shows adequate physiological reserve. Monitoring ensures continued stability. This reflects a temporary adjustment period. ##
Q670. Answer: D
Explanation: Individualized teaching addresses specific gaps in knowledge and confidence. Reinforcement ensures understanding of key concepts. Providing support helps reduce anxiety. Clear instructions improve patient safety. Resources assist with limited support systems. This approach ensures readiness for safe discharge. ##
Q671. Answer: C
Explanation: Early breastfeeding stimulates the release of prolactin and oxytocin. These hormones support milk production and ejection. Initiating feeding early improves long-term lactation success. It also promotes bonding between mother and infant. Early feeding supports neonatal glucose stability. This practice is recommended for optimal outcomes. ##
Q672. Answer: B
Explanation: Hypocalcemia affects neuromuscular function in newborns. This can lead to twitching or jitteriness. Early recognition is important to prevent complications. Calcium supplementation may be required. Monitoring ensures normalization of levels. This condition requires prompt management. ##
Q673. Answer: B
Explanation: Irregular feeding can lead to milk accumulation and discomfort. Encouraging consistent feeding helps maintain milk flow. This prevents engorgement and reduces pain. Proper latch and positioning should also be addressed. Monitoring ensures symptom improvement. This supports effective breastfeeding management. ##
Q674. Answer: D
Explanation: Yellow discoloration indicates elevated bilirubin levels. This condition is known as neonatal jaundice. Mild lethargy and poor feeding are common associated findings. Early assessment determines severity. Treatment may include phototherapy. Monitoring prevents complications such as bilirubin toxicity. ##
Q675. Answer: B
Explanation: Fever may indicate infection in the postpartum period. Early detection is important for treatment. Patients should be educated to monitor temperature. Prompt reporting ensures timely intervention. Monitoring helps prevent complications. This supports safe postpartum recovery. ##
Q676. Answer: B
Explanation: These symptoms indicate difficulty with breathing and oxygenation. Grunting and retractions show increased effort. Low oxygen saturation confirms inadequate gas exchange. Immediate intervention is required. Monitoring guides treatment. Early care improves outcomes. ##
Q677. Answer: D
Explanation: Breast milk should be stored according to established guidelines. Refrigeration helps maintain quality and safety. Proper storage prevents bacterial growth. Clean containers should be used. Education ensures safe feeding practices. This helps preserve nutritional benefits for the infant. ##
Q678. Answer: C

Explanation: Hand hygiene is essential to prevent infection transmission. Failure to perform it compromises patient safety. Reporting ensures accountability and adherence to standards. Following institutional policy is required. Ignoring the issue increases risk of infection. This action supports quality care and safety. ##

Q679. Answer: D

Explanation: Some newborns require minimal assistance during transition. Rapid improvement indicates mild difficulty. Weak initial responses are common. Recovery with simple interventions shows adequate reserve. Monitoring ensures stability continues. This reflects a temporary adjustment period. ##

Q680. Answer: D

Explanation: Repeated individualized education reinforces important concepts. Addressing concerns improves patient confidence. Providing support helps reduce anxiety. Clear instructions ensure safe newborn care. Resources assist with limited support systems. This approach ensures readiness for discharge. ##

Q681. Answer: A

Explanation: Prolactin is responsible for milk production in the mammary glands. Its release is stimulated by infant suckling. Frequent breastfeeding maintains elevated prolactin levels. This supports ongoing milk supply. Without stimulation, levels decrease and production declines. Consistent feeding is essential for sustained lactation. ##

Q682. Answer: B

Explanation: Hypothermia increases metabolic demand in newborns. This leads to rapid glucose consumption. As glucose levels fall, hypoglycemia develops. Maintaining warmth helps prevent this complication. Early detection is essential for management. Monitoring ensures stabilization of metabolic status. ##

Q683. Answer: B

Explanation: Poor latch is a common cause of nipple trauma and ineffective feeding. Assessing positioning helps ensure proper attachment. Correct latch reduces pain and improves milk transfer. Continued breastfeeding supports healing when technique is corrected. Education is essential for success. Early intervention prevents further complications. ##

Q684. Answer: D

Explanation: Hypoglycemia affects neurological function in newborns. Symptoms include tremors and irritability. Poor feeding is also a common sign. Early recognition is critical to prevent complications. Treatment includes feeding or glucose administration. Monitoring ensures stabilization of glucose levels. ##

Q685. Answer: D

Explanation: Visual disturbances may indicate serious conditions such as hypertension. Early recognition is essential for prompt treatment. These symptoms should not be ignored. Patients must be educated on danger signs. Prompt reporting improves outcomes. Monitoring ensures patient safety. ##

Q686. Answer: B

Explanation: These signs indicate increased work of breathing. Grunting and retractions show respiratory compromise. Low oxygen saturation confirms inadequate oxygenation. Immediate intervention is required. Monitoring guides management. Early care improves neonatal outcomes. ##

Q687. Answer: C

Explanation: Frequent and consistent pumping mimics infant feeding patterns. This helps maintain prolactin levels and milk production. Skipping sessions can decrease supply. Night pumping may also be necessary early on. Education supports sustained lactation. This approach ensures adequate milk availability. ##

Q688. Answer: D

Explanation: Medication safety requires strict adherence to protocols. Bypassing checks increases risk of patient harm. Reporting ensures accountability and prevention of future errors. Following institutional policy is essential. Ignoring the issue compromises safety. This action supports a culture of safe practice. ##

Q689. Answer: A

Explanation: Some newborns require minimal assistance during transition. Rapid improvement indicates mild adaptation difficulty. Weak initial responses are not uncommon. Recovery with simple interventions shows adequate physiological reserve. Monitoring ensures continued stability. This reflects a temporary adjustment process. ##

Q690. Answer: D

Explanation: Repeated individualized education helps address persistent knowledge gaps. Tailored teaching improves understanding and confidence. Emotional support reduces anxiety and promotes readiness. Clear instructions ensure safe newborn care at home. Providing resources supports patients with limited support systems. This approach ensures a safe and effective discharge process. ##

Q691. Answer: D

Explanation: Colostrum is the first milk produced after delivery. It is thick and rich in antibodies that protect the newborn. This milk provides essential immune support during early life. It is produced in small amounts but is highly concentrated. Colostrum helps prepare the infant's digestive system. It gradually transitions into mature milk. ##

Q692. Answer: D

Explanation: Hypocalcemia can affect neuromuscular stability in newborns. Severe cases may lead to seizure-like activity. Early recognition is important to prevent complications. Calcium supplementation is often required. Monitoring ensures normalization of calcium levels. Prompt treatment supports neurological stability. ##

Q693. Answer: B

Explanation: Ineffective latch is a common cause of nipple damage and poor milk transfer. Reassessing positioning ensures proper attachment to the breast. Correct technique reduces trauma and improves feeding efficiency. Continued breastfeeding supports healing when latch is corrected. Education enhances maternal confidence. Early correction prevents worsening symptoms. ##

Q694. Answer: A

Explanation: Hypoglycemia affects neurological function in newborns. Symptoms include lethargy, weak cry, and poor feeding. Low glucose levels reduce energy supply to the brain. Early detection is critical to prevent long-term complications. Treatment involves feeding or glucose administration. Monitoring ensures stabilization of glucose levels. ##

Q695. Answer: D

Explanation: Sudden severe abdominal pain may indicate serious complications such as internal bleeding. Early recognition is essential for prompt intervention. This symptom should not be ignored. Patients must be educated on warning signs before discharge. Immediate evaluation can prevent worsening conditions. Monitoring ensures patient safety. ##

Q696. Answer: C

Explanation: Persistent respiratory symptoms indicate compromised lung function. Tachypnea and retractions show increased effort to breathe. Low oxygen saturation confirms inadequate gas exchange. Continued support and monitoring are required. Early intervention improves outcomes. This condition requires prompt medical management. ##

Q697. Answer: D

Explanation: Irregular pumping can lead to decreased milk production. Consistent stimulation is required to maintain prolactin levels. Reinforcing a regular schedule helps restore supply. Frequent emptying of the breasts supports ongoing production. Education encourages adherence to routine. This approach improves lactation outcomes. ##

Q698. Answer: A

Explanation: Patient identification is a critical safety step in medication administration. Failure to verify identity increases the risk of serious errors. Reporting ensures accountability and system improvement. Following institutional policy supports safe practice. Ignoring the issue compromises patient safety. This action promotes a culture of quality care. ##

Q699. Answer: C

Explanation: Some newborns experience mild difficulty during initial adaptation. Rapid improvement with minimal intervention indicates adequate physiological reserve. Weak initial responses are not uncommon. Recovery with simple measures confirms stable transition. Monitoring ensures continued progress. This reflects a temporary adjustment period. ##

Q700. Answer: C

Explanation: Repeated structured education helps reinforce key concepts. Addressing persistent gaps improves patient understanding. Emotional support reduces anxiety and increases confidence. Clear and repeated instructions ensure safe care at home. Providing resources supports patients with limited support systems. This approach ensures readiness for discharge and patient safety. ## Question (701-750)

Question (701-750)

Q701. The component of breast milk that promotes healthy gut flora in the newborn is what?
(A) Mineral electrolyte balance
(B) Protein enzyme structure
(C) Fatty acid content
(D) Oligosaccharide compounds

Q702. A newborn experiencing hypothermia may show which behavioral sign?
(A) Vigorous feeding pattern
(B) Strong crying behavior
(C) Increased alertness state
(D) Lethargy or decreased activity

Q703. A postpartum patient reports that milk supply appears to be decreasing after spacing out feeding sessions due to fatigue and irregular scheduling, and expresses concern about meeting infant nutritional needs; what is the most appropriate nursing intervention?
(A) Encourage more frequent feeding or pumping
(B) Reduce feeding sessions further
(C) Switch entirely to formula
(D) Stop breastfeeding temporarily

Q704. A newborn develops high-pitched crying, irritability, tremors, and poor feeding within hours of birth, and laboratory testing reveals low calcium levels; what condition is most likely present?
(A) Neonatal hypoglycemia
(B) Respiratory distress syndrome
(C) Neonatal infection process
(D) Neonatal hypocalcemia state

Q705. A postpartum patient is taught to recognize signs of hemorrhage; which symptom should prompt immediate action?
(A) Occasional mood swings
(B) Breast fullness sensation
(C) Mild fatigue feeling
(D) Saturating pads rapidly

Q706. A newborn presents with persistent tachypnea, nasal flaring, intercostal retractions, and decreased oxygen saturation despite initial interventions; what condition is most likely present?
(A) Respiratory distress condition
(B) Thermoregulation imbalance
(C) Feeding difficulty issue
(D) Normal transition process

Q707. A postpartum patient exclusively pumping breast milk reports declining output after reducing nighttime pumping sessions and extending intervals between sessions due to fatigue; what is the most appropriate nursing recommendation?
(A) Eliminate additional sessions
(B) Reinforce frequent pumping schedule
(C) Avoid consistent expression
(D) Stop pumping at night

Q708. A nurse identifies that a colleague is documenting care that was not performed for a postpartum patient, raising concerns about ethical practice; what is the most appropriate action?
(A) Confront without reporting
(B) Ignore the situation

(C) Report according to ethical guidelines
(D) Document similar behavior

Q709. A newborn demonstrates irregular respirations, weak cry, and decreased tone immediately after delivery but responds quickly to stimulation, warming, and airway positioning, showing improvement within minutes; what does this indicate about neonatal transition?

(A) Circulatory collapse
(B) Severe respiratory failure
(C) Mild transitional difficulty
(D) Neurological impairment

Q710. A postpartum patient preparing for discharge expresses concerns about breastfeeding challenges, identifying newborn complications, safe sleep practices, and managing care independently due to lack of support, while also showing persistent anxiety and misunderstanding of instructions despite repeated teaching; the nurse reassesses readiness and identifies ongoing deficits. What is the most appropriate nursing action in this situation?

(A) Refer without further guidance
(B) Delay discharge without explanation
(C) Avoid addressing concerns
(D) Provide structured repeated teaching with support

Q711. The nutrient in breast milk primarily responsible for providing energy to the newborn is what?

(A) Enzyme protein structure
(B) Lactose carbohydrate source
(C) Mineral electrolyte level
(D) Immunoglobulin antibody type

Q712. A newborn with hypoglycemia may also present with which cardiovascular sign?

(A) Bradycardia stability
(B) Tachycardia response
(C) Normal heart rhythm
(D) Elevated blood pressure

Q713. A postpartum patient reports decreased milk supply after skipping several feeding sessions due to fatigue and discomfort, and expresses concern about infant intake and satisfaction; what is the most appropriate nursing intervention?

(A) Switch completely to formula
(B) Stop breastfeeding temporarily
(C) Reinforce frequent feeding or pumping
(D) Continue skipping feeding sessions

Q714. A newborn develops jitteriness, irritability, and poor feeding within the first hours after birth, and laboratory results reveal low calcium levels; what condition is most likely present?

(A) Neonatal hypoglycemia
(B) Respiratory distress syndrome
(C) Neonatal hypocalcemia state
(D) Neonatal infection process

Q715. A postpartum patient is instructed on warning signs of complications; which symptom requires immediate medical attention?

(A) Breast fullness sensation
(B) Mild fatigue feeling
(C) Occasional mood changes
(D) Sudden onset chest tightness

Q716. A newborn presents with rapid breathing, nasal flaring, intercostal retractions, and decreased oxygen saturation shortly after birth despite initial stabilization efforts; what condition is most likely present?
(A) Respiratory distress condition
(B) Feeding difficulty issue
(C) Thermoregulation imbalance
(D) Normal transition process
Q717. A postpartum patient exclusively pumping breast milk reports declining production after reducing pumping sessions and extending intervals due to work demands and fatigue; what is the most appropriate nursing recommendation?
(A) Reduce pumping sessions further
(B) Stop pumping at night
(C) Avoid scheduled expression
(D) Increase pumping frequency consistently
Q718. A nurse observes a colleague bypassing hand hygiene before caring for a newborn, increasing the risk of infection transmission; what is the most appropriate professional action?
(A) Ignore the behavior
(B) Document similar practice
(C) Confront without escalation
(D) Report according to protocol
Q719. A newborn demonstrates weak respiratory effort, decreased tone, and delayed crying at birth but shows rapid improvement after stimulation, warming, and airway support within a few minutes; what does this indicate about neonatal transition?
(A) Severe respiratory failure
(B) Neurological impairment
(C) Circulatory collapse
(D) Mild transitional difficulty
Q720. A postpartum patient preparing for discharge expresses concerns about breastfeeding effectiveness, recognizing newborn complications, safe sleep practices, and managing care independently due to limited support, while also showing anxiety and repeated misunderstanding of instructions despite multiple teaching sessions; the nurse reassesses readiness and identifies persistent learning gaps. What is the most appropriate nursing action in this situation?
(A) Provide reinforced individualized teaching and support
(B) Avoid addressing concerns
(C) Delay discharge without explanation
(D) Refer without further education
Q721. The reflex that helps a newborn locate the breast for feeding is what?
(A) Babinski reflex sign
(B) Rooting reflex response
(C) Tonic neck reflex
(D) Moro reflex reaction
Q722. A newborn with hypothermia may develop which respiratory change due to increased metabolic demand?
(A) Stable oxygen requirement
(B) Decreased respiratory effort
(C) Reduced breathing rate
(D) Increased oxygen consumption

Q723. A postpartum patient reports that the infant frequently falls asleep shortly after latching and feeds for very short periods, resulting in continued breast fullness and concern about milk transfer; what is the most appropriate nursing intervention?
(A) Encourage effective feeding techniques
(B) Stop breastfeeding temporarily
(C) Reduce feeding frequency
(D) Switch to formula feeding
Q724. A newborn presents with irritability, tremors, and high-pitched cry shortly after birth, and laboratory findings reveal low blood glucose levels; what condition is most likely present?
(A) Neonatal hypocalcemia
(B) Neonatal infection process
(C) Neonatal hypoglycemia state
(D) Respiratory distress syndrome
Q725. A postpartum patient is instructed on signs of infection; which symptom should be reported immediately?
(A) Breast fullness sensation
(B) Occasional mood swings
(C) Mild fatigue feeling
(D) Persistent high fever
Q726. A newborn develops rapid breathing, nasal flaring, and chest retractions with decreasing oxygen saturation despite initial stabilization efforts; what condition is most likely present?
(A) Feeding difficulty issue
(B) Respiratory distress condition
(C) Normal transition process
(D) Thermoregulation imbalance
Q727. A postpartum patient who is exclusively pumping reports reduced milk output after inconsistent pumping intervals due to fatigue and schedule changes, and seeks advice to restore supply; what is the most appropriate recommendation?
(A) Maintain consistent frequent pumping
(B) Stop pumping temporarily
(C) Reduce pumping sessions
(D) Avoid scheduled expression
Q728. A nurse observes a colleague discussing confidential patient information in a public setting where others can hear; what is the most appropriate professional action?
(A) Document similar actions
(B) Ignore the behavior
(C) Report confidentiality breach
(D) Participate in discussion
Q729. A newborn demonstrates weak cry, decreased tone, and irregular respirations immediately after birth but responds rapidly to stimulation, warming, and airway positioning within a few minutes; what does this indicate about neonatal adaptation?
(A) Circulatory collapse
(B) Severe respiratory failure
(C) Neurological impairment
(D) Mild transitional difficulty
Q730. A postpartum patient preparing for discharge reports concerns about breastfeeding success, identifying newborn complications, safe sleep practices, and managing care independently due to limited support, while also demonstrating anxiety and misunderstanding of instructions despite

repeated teaching sessions; the nurse reassesses readiness and identifies ongoing gaps. What is the most appropriate nursing action in this situation?
(A) Avoid addressing concerns
(B) Delay discharge without explanation
(C) Refer without further guidance
(D) Provide structured repeated teaching and support
Q731. The reflex that causes a newborn to grasp an object placed in the palm is what?
(A) Moro reflex reaction
(B) Palmar grasp reflex
(C) Rooting reflex response
(D) Babinski reflex sign
Q732. A newborn exposed to prolonged cold stress may develop which acid-base imbalance?
(A) Metabolic alkalosis state
(B) Respiratory acidosis state
(C) Metabolic acidosis condition
(D) Respiratory alkalosis state
Q733. A postpartum patient reports difficulty with breastfeeding due to the infant slipping off the breast frequently and ineffective sucking, resulting in prolonged feeding times and continued breast fullness; what is the most appropriate nursing intervention?
(A) Reduce feeding frequency
(B) Switch to formula feeding
(C) Stop breastfeeding temporarily
(D) Assess latch and positioning technique
Q734. A newborn presents with jitteriness, irritability, poor feeding, and laboratory results showing low blood glucose levels shortly after birth; what condition is most likely present?
(A) Neonatal hypoglycemia state
(B) Neonatal infection process
(C) Neonatal hypocalcemia
(D) Respiratory distress syndrome
Q735. A postpartum patient is educated on warning signs before discharge; which symptom requires immediate medical evaluation?
(A) Occasional mood swings
(B) Sudden severe headache
(C) Breast fullness sensation
(D) Mild fatigue feeling
Q736. A newborn develops persistent tachypnea, nasal flaring, and intercostal retractions with decreasing oxygen saturation despite initial stabilization measures; what condition is most likely present?
(A) Feeding difficulty issue
(B) Respiratory distress condition
(C) Thermoregulation imbalance
(D) Normal transition process
Q737. A postpartum patient exclusively pumping breast milk reports declining production after irregular pumping intervals and skipped sessions due to fatigue and work demands; what is the most appropriate nursing recommendation?
(A) Reinforce consistent pumping schedule
(B) Reduce pumping sessions further
(C) Avoid nighttime expression

(D) Stop pumping temporarily

Q738. A nurse observes a colleague failing to maintain sterile technique during a postpartum procedure, increasing infection risk; what is the most appropriate professional action?

(A) Confront without escalation
(B) Report according to protocol
(C) Document similar practice
(D) Ignore the behavior

Q739. A newborn demonstrates weak cry, decreased tone, and irregular respirations immediately after birth but responds rapidly to stimulation, warming, and airway support within minutes; what does this indicate about neonatal adaptation?

(A) Severe respiratory failure
(B) Mild transitional difficulty
(C) Circulatory collapse
(D) Neurological impairment

Q740. A postpartum patient preparing for discharge expresses concerns about breastfeeding success, recognizing newborn complications, safe sleep practices, and managing care independently due to limited support, while also demonstrating anxiety and repeated misunderstanding despite prior teaching; the nurse reassesses readiness and identifies persistent knowledge gaps. What is the most appropriate nursing action in this situation?

(A) Delay discharge without explanation
(B) Refer without additional teaching
(C) Provide structured repeated education and support
(D) Avoid addressing concerns

Q741. The reflex that causes extension of the toes when the sole of the foot is stroked is what?

(A) Babinski reflex response
(B) Rooting reflex action
(C) Palmar grasp reflex
(D) Moro reflex reaction

Q742. A newborn experiencing cold stress may develop which respiratory complication due to increased oxygen demand?

(A) Decreased oxygen use
(B) Stable respiratory rate
(C) Normal breathing pattern
(D) Respiratory distress condition

Q743. A postpartum patient reports that the infant frequently slips off the breast and feeds for long periods without satisfaction, leading to breast fullness and discomfort between feeds; what is the most appropriate nursing intervention?

(A) Evaluate latch and positioning technique
(B) Switch completely to formula
(C) Stop breastfeeding temporarily
(D) Reduce feeding frequency

Q744. A newborn exhibits poor feeding, lethargy, hypotonia, and weak cry within hours after birth, and blood glucose testing confirms low levels; what condition is most likely present?

(A) Neonatal jaundice condition
(B) Neonatal hypoglycemia condition
(C) Neonatal hypocalcemia condition
(D) Neonatal sepsis condition

Q745. A postpartum patient reports sudden onset of severe pelvic pain accompanied by heavy bleeding and passage of large clots several days after delivery; what complication should be suspected?
(A) Normal uterine involution
(B) Postpartum mood change
(C) Breast engorgement issue
(D) Secondary postpartum hemorrhage
Q746. A newborn presents with central cyanosis, grunting respirations, and persistent oxygen desaturation despite initial oxygen therapy shortly after birth; what is the most likely condition?
(A) Severe respiratory distress condition
(B) Feeding coordination problem
(C) Normal transitional adaptation
(D) Mild thermoregulation issue
Q747. A postpartum patient who is breastfeeding reports decreased milk production after supplementing frequently with formula and skipping multiple breastfeeding sessions over several days; what is the most appropriate nursing recommendation?
(A) Stop breastfeeding completely
(B) Resume frequent direct breastfeeding
(C) Limit infant feeding attempts
(D) Increase formula supplementation
Q748. A nurse notices that a colleague intentionally omitted documenting a medication error involving a newborn patient, raising serious ethical concerns; what is the most appropriate professional action?
(A) Report the incident through proper channels
(B) Confront privately without reporting
(C) Document similar behavior
(D) Ignore since no harm occurred
Q749. A newborn shows decreased tone, minimal respiratory effort, and delayed crying at birth but responds promptly to stimulation and warming with rapid improvement in vital signs; what does this indicate about neonatal adaptation?
(A) Mild transitional adjustment
(B) Cardiovascular collapse
(C) Severe respiratory failure
(D) Permanent neurological deficit
Q750. A postpartum patient preparing for discharge expresses multiple concerns including difficulty breastfeeding, inability to recognize early newborn illness, uncertainty about safe sleep positioning, and lack of family support, while also demonstrating anxiety and confusion despite prior teaching; the nurse identifies that the patient is not fully ready for independent care. What is the most appropriate nursing action in this situation?
(A) Avoid reinforcing previously taught content
(B) Proceed with discharge without further teaching
(C) Provide intensive individualized discharge teaching and resources
(D) Refer patient without additional instruction

Answer Key and Explanation (701-750)

Q701. Answer: D

Explanation: Oligosaccharides in breast milk support the growth of beneficial bacteria. These compounds help establish healthy gut flora in the newborn. They also prevent harmful pathogens from attaching to the intestinal lining. This contributes to improved digestive health. Breast milk components work together to enhance immunity. This supports long-term gastrointestinal development. ##

Q702. Answer: D

Explanation: Hypothermia reduces metabolic activity in newborns. This leads to lethargy and decreased responsiveness. Early detection is essential to prevent complications. Maintaining warmth is critical for stabilization. Monitoring ensures improvement in condition. Prompt intervention supports neonatal safety. ##

Q703. Answer: A

Explanation: Decreased stimulation leads to reduced prolactin levels. This results in decreased milk production. Increasing feeding or pumping frequency helps restore supply. Consistent breast emptying supports ongoing production. Education encourages adherence to routine. This approach improves lactation success. ##

Q704. Answer: D

Explanation: Hypocalcemia affects neuromuscular function in newborns. Symptoms include irritability and tremors. A high-pitched cry may also be present. Early detection is essential to prevent complications. Treatment includes calcium supplementation. Monitoring ensures normalization of calcium levels. ##

Q705. Answer: D

Explanation: Rapid saturation of pads indicates excessive bleeding. This may suggest postpartum hemorrhage. Immediate intervention is required to prevent complications. Patients must be educated on recognizing abnormal bleeding. Prompt reporting ensures timely care. Monitoring supports patient safety. ##

Q706. Answer: A

Explanation: Persistent respiratory symptoms indicate compromised lung function. Tachypnea and retractions show increased effort to breathe. Low oxygen saturation confirms inadequate gas exchange. Ongoing support is required. Monitoring guides treatment decisions. Early intervention improves outcomes. ##

Q707. Answer: B

Explanation: Reduced pumping frequency leads to decreased milk production. Prolactin levels depend on regular stimulation. Reinforcing frequent sessions helps restore supply. Nighttime pumping may be important early on. Education supports adherence to routine. This approach improves lactation outcomes. ##

Q708. Answer: C

Explanation: Falsification of documentation is a serious ethical violation. It compromises patient safety and legal accountability. Reporting ensures corrective action is taken. Following professional guidelines is essential. Ignoring the issue can lead to further harm. This action upholds ethical standards in care. ##

Q709. Answer: C

Explanation: Some newborns require minimal support during transition. Rapid improvement indicates mild adaptation difficulty. Initial weak responses are not uncommon. Recovery with simple interventions shows adequate physiological reserve. Monitoring ensures continued stability. This reflects a temporary adjustment phase. ##

Q710. Answer: D

Explanation: Structured repeated teaching reinforces key concepts effectively. Addressing ongoing concerns improves patient confidence. Emotional support reduces anxiety levels. Clear instructions ensure safe newborn care practices. Resources assist patients with limited support systems. This approach ensures readiness for safe discharge. ##

Q711. Answer: B

Explanation: Lactose is the primary carbohydrate in breast milk and provides energy. It supports brain development and growth. Lactose also aids in calcium absorption. This nutrient is essential for metabolic processes. Adequate intake ensures proper development. Breast milk composition is designed to meet infant energy needs. ##

Q712. Answer: B

Explanation: Hypoglycemia can stimulate a stress response in newborns. This may lead to tachycardia as the body attempts to compensate. The increased heart rate reflects metabolic imbalance. Early detection is essential to prevent worsening. Treatment includes feeding or glucose administration. Monitoring ensures stabilization of vital signs. ##

Q713. Answer: C

Explanation: Skipping feedings reduces stimulation needed for milk production. Prolactin levels decrease without regular demand. Reinforcing frequent feeding helps restore supply. Consistent breast emptying supports ongoing production. Education encourages adherence to feeding schedules. This approach improves lactation success. ##

Q714. Answer: C

Explanation: Hypocalcemia affects neuromuscular stability in newborns. Symptoms include jitteriness and irritability. Poor feeding may also occur. Early recognition is important to prevent complications. Treatment includes calcium supplementation. Monitoring ensures normalization of calcium levels. ##

Q715. Answer: D

Explanation: Chest tightness may indicate a serious condition such as pulmonary embolism. Postpartum patients are at increased risk for thromboembolic events. Immediate evaluation is essential. Early intervention can prevent life-threatening complications. Patients must be educated on recognizing warning signs. Prompt reporting ensures timely care. ##

Q716. Answer: A

Explanation: These signs indicate impaired respiratory function. Rapid breathing and retractions show increased effort. Decreased oxygen saturation confirms inadequate gas exchange. Immediate intervention is required. Monitoring guides further management. Early treatment improves neonatal outcomes. ##

Q717. Answer: D

Explanation: Milk production depends on regular stimulation. Reduced pumping leads to decreased prolactin levels. Increasing frequency helps restore supply. Consistent intervals are essential for maintaining production. Education supports adherence to routine. This approach improves lactation outcomes. ##

Q718. Answer: D

Explanation: Hand hygiene is critical for preventing infection in vulnerable populations. Newborns are particularly at risk. Reporting ensures adherence to safety standards. Following institutional protocol supports quality care. Ignoring the issue increases risk of harm. This action promotes patient safety. ##

Q719. Answer: D

Explanation: Some newborns require minimal assistance during transition. Rapid improvement indicates mild difficulty. Initial weak responses are not uncommon. Recovery with simple interventions shows adequate reserve. Monitoring ensures continued stability. This reflects a temporary adaptation phase. ##

Q720. Answer: A

Explanation: Reinforced individualized teaching addresses persistent knowledge gaps. Tailored education improves understanding and confidence. Emotional support reduces anxiety and promotes readiness. Clear instructions ensure safe newborn care practices. Providing resources helps compensate for limited support. This approach ensures a safe and effective discharge process. ##

Q721. Answer: B

Explanation: The rooting reflex helps the newborn turn toward a stimulus on the cheek. This allows the infant to locate the breast for feeding. It is an essential reflex for successful breastfeeding. The reflex is present at birth and gradually disappears. Assessment of this reflex helps evaluate neurological function. It supports effective feeding behavior in early life. ##

Q722. Answer: D

Explanation: Hypothermia increases metabolic demands in newborns. This leads to increased oxygen consumption. The body attempts to generate heat through metabolism. As a result, respiratory workload increases. Early warming helps reduce oxygen demand. Monitoring ensures stabilization of respiratory status. ##

Q723. Answer: A

Explanation: Ineffective feeding can lead to inadequate milk transfer. Encouraging proper positioning and stimulation helps maintain feeding. Keeping the infant awake during feeds improves intake. Frequent feeding prevents engorgement. Education supports successful breastfeeding. Monitoring ensures improvement in feeding patterns. ##

Q724. Answer: C

Explanation: Hypoglycemia affects neurological stability in newborns. Symptoms include tremors and irritability. A high-pitched cry may also occur. Early detection is essential to prevent complications. Treatment includes feeding or glucose administration. Monitoring ensures stabilization of glucose levels. ##

Q725. Answer: D

Explanation: Persistent fever may indicate infection in the postpartum period. Early recognition is essential for treatment. Patients should be educated to monitor temperature changes. Prompt reporting ensures timely intervention. Monitoring helps prevent complications. This supports safe postpartum recovery. ##

Q726. Answer: B

Explanation: These signs indicate increased work of breathing. Decreased oxygen saturation confirms inadequate gas exchange. Persistent symptoms suggest respiratory distress. Immediate intervention is required. Monitoring guides treatment decisions. Early management improves neonatal outcomes. ##

Q727. Answer: A

Explanation: Inconsistent pumping reduces stimulation needed for milk production. Maintaining frequent sessions helps restore prolactin levels. Consistent breast emptying supports ongoing supply. Education encourages adherence to routine. Monitoring ensures improvement in output. This approach supports effective lactation management. ##

Q728. Answer: C

Explanation: Discussing patient information publicly violates confidentiality. Protecting privacy is a legal and ethical responsibility. Reporting ensures accountability and prevention of future incidents. Following institutional policies is required. Ignoring the issue compromises patient trust. This action supports professional standards. ##

Q729. Answer: D

Explanation: Some newborns require minimal support during transition. Rapid improvement indicates mild adaptation difficulty. Weak initial responses are common. Recovery with simple interventions shows adequate physiological reserve. Monitoring ensures continued stability. This reflects a temporary adjustment phase. ##

Q730. Answer: D
Explanation: Structured repeated teaching helps reinforce essential information. Addressing concerns improves patient confidence. Emotional support reduces anxiety levels. Clear instructions ensure safe newborn care. Providing resources supports patients with limited support. This approach ensures readiness for discharge. ##
Q731. Answer: B
Explanation: The palmar grasp reflex causes the infant to close the hand around an object. It is present at birth and indicates neurological integrity. This reflex helps assess motor development. It gradually disappears as voluntary control develops. Evaluation is part of newborn assessment. It reflects normal neurological function. ##
Q732. Answer: C
Explanation: Cold stress increases metabolic demand and oxygen consumption. When oxygen is insufficient, anaerobic metabolism occurs. This leads to lactic acid accumulation. As a result, metabolic acidosis develops. Early warming prevents this complication. Monitoring ensures correction of acid-base balance. ##
Q733. Answer: D
Explanation: Ineffective latch leads to poor milk transfer and prolonged feeding. Assessing positioning helps improve attachment. Correct latch enhances feeding efficiency. Continued breastfeeding supports milk supply. Education improves maternal confidence. Early correction prevents complications such as engorgement. ##
Q734. Answer: A
Explanation: Hypoglycemia affects neurological function in newborns. Symptoms include jitteriness and irritability. Poor feeding is also common. Early detection is critical to prevent complications. Treatment includes feeding or glucose administration. Monitoring ensures stabilization of glucose levels. ##
Q735. Answer: B
Explanation: A sudden severe headache may indicate hypertensive complications. Postpartum patients are at risk for conditions like preeclampsia. Early recognition is essential for treatment. Patients must be educated on warning signs. Prompt reporting ensures timely intervention. Monitoring supports patient safety. ##
Q736. Answer: B
Explanation: These signs indicate impaired respiratory function. Tachypnea and retractions reflect increased effort. Decreased oxygen saturation confirms poor gas exchange. Immediate intervention is required. Monitoring guides further management. Early treatment improves outcomes. ##
Q737. Answer: A
Explanation: Irregular pumping reduces stimulation needed for milk production. Consistent scheduling helps maintain prolactin levels. Frequent emptying supports ongoing milk supply. Education encourages adherence to routine. Monitoring ensures improvement in output. This approach supports successful lactation management. ##
Q738. Answer: B
Explanation: Maintaining sterile technique is essential to prevent infection. Failure to follow protocols increases patient risk. Reporting ensures corrective action is taken. Following institutional policy supports safe practice. Ignoring the issue compromises patient safety. This action promotes quality care. ##
Q739. Answer: B
Explanation: Some newborns require minimal support during transition. Rapid improvement indicates mild adaptation difficulty. Initial weak responses are common. Recovery with simple measures shows adequate physiological reserve. Monitoring ensures continued stability. This reflects a temporary adjustment phase. ##

Q740. Answer: C
Explanation: Structured repeated education reinforces key concepts effectively. Addressing concerns improves patient understanding. Emotional support reduces anxiety levels. Clear instructions ensure safe newborn care. Providing resources helps patients with limited support. This approach ensures readiness for discharge and safe care at home. ##
Q741. Answer: A
Explanation: The Babinski reflex is elicited by stroking the sole of the foot. This causes the toes to fan outward and extend. It is a normal finding in newborns due to immature nervous systems. The reflex disappears as neurological development progresses. Assessment helps evaluate neurological function. It is an important part of newborn examination. ##
Q742. Answer: D
Explanation: Cold stress increases metabolic demand and oxygen consumption. This can lead to respiratory distress if oxygen supply is insufficient. The newborn may show signs such as tachypnea. Early warming reduces oxygen demand. Monitoring ensures respiratory stability. Prompt intervention prevents complications. ##
Q743. Answer: A
Explanation: Poor latch results in ineffective milk transfer. Evaluating positioning helps ensure proper attachment. Correct latch improves feeding efficiency and reduces discomfort. Continued breastfeeding supports milk production. Education enhances maternal confidence. Early correction prevents complications such as engorgement. ##
Q744. Answer: B
Explanation: Hypoglycemia leads to decreased energy availability for the brain. This results in lethargy, poor feeding, and hypotonia. A weak cry may also be observed. Early identification is essential to prevent neurological damage. Treatment includes prompt feeding or glucose administration. Monitoring ensures stabilization and prevents recurrence. ##
Q745. Answer: D
Explanation: Secondary postpartum hemorrhage occurs after the first 24 hours postpartum. It is characterized by heavy bleeding and clot passage. Severe pelvic pain may accompany uterine complications. Immediate evaluation is required to prevent shock. Causes may include retained placental tissue or infection. Early intervention improves maternal outcomes. ##
Q746. Answer: A
Explanation: Central cyanosis indicates inadequate oxygenation. Grunting respirations suggest increased effort to maintain airway pressure. Persistent desaturation despite oxygen therapy signals significant respiratory compromise. Immediate advanced support may be required. Early diagnosis is critical for management. Continuous monitoring ensures stabilization. ##
Q747. Answer: B
Explanation: Frequent breastfeeding stimulates prolactin release, which maintains milk production. Skipping sessions reduces demand and decreases supply. Resuming regular breastfeeding helps restore production. Direct feeding is more effective than supplementation for stimulation. Education supports adherence to feeding routines. This approach promotes successful lactation. ##
Q748. Answer: A
Explanation: Failure to report errors violates ethical and professional standards. Documentation ensures transparency and patient safety. Reporting allows system review and prevention of future incidents. Even if no harm occurred, accountability is required. Following institutional policy is essential. This action upholds professional integrity. ##
Q749. Answer: A
Explanation: Mild transitional difficulty is common in some newborns. Initial depression may occur but resolves quickly with minimal intervention. Rapid response indicates adequate physiological reserve.

Continued monitoring ensures stability. No advanced intervention is typically required. This reflects normal adaptation variation. ##

Q750. Answer: C

Explanation: Intensive individualized teaching addresses multiple knowledge gaps. Reinforcement improves understanding and retention of critical information. Addressing emotional concerns reduces anxiety and promotes confidence. Providing resources supports patients with limited social support. Ensuring readiness is essential for safe home care. This approach promotes positive maternal and newborn outcomes. ##

Made in United States
Orlando, FL
05 November 2026

90229886R00122